GRASP

Ursula Fleming was born into a Catholic family in Liverpool in 1930, her mother being a doctor and her father a surgeon. At the age of six she was diagnosed as a musician, and won her first festival two years later. At fifteen, when her father died, she gave up Catholicism and her musical training, turning instead to the study of relaxation at Crichton Royal Hospital, Dumfries.

She has worked at the Oxford Regional Pain Relief Unit, Sobell House, Oxford, the Royal Free Hospital, London and also in Harley Street. She has lectured on pain control on both radio and television, and has produced two cassettes on the subject.

GRASPING THE NETTLE

A Positive Approach to Pain

URSULA FLEMING

Collins
FOUNT PAPERBACKS

First published in Great Britain by
Fount Paperbacks, London in 1990

Copyright © Ursula Fleming 1990

Typeset by Avocet Robinson, Buckingham

Printed and bound in Great Britain by
William Collins Sons & Co. Ltd, Glasgow

This book is dedicated to
the memory of Marco Pallis,
of Dr W. Mayer-Gross
and of Professor John Hay

Acknowledgements for their help to my children Adam, Suella, Barnaby John and Rory.

To my sisters Anne and Mary.

To Father Conrad Peplar OP and to Lord Craigmyle.

And to Professor Kenneth Hobbs and the staff in the Academic Department of Surgery and on Jex Blake ward at the Royal Free Hospital, London, for their kindness, open-mindedness and support.

*

CONTENTS

Foreword

The nettle to grasp is that of pain and suffering. We are
not helpless in the face of pain, for we can survive and
overcome it. We have an innate power of adaptation to
the world around us but we are so convinced that our only
option is to try to avoid pain that we rarely consider any
alternative.

We don't consciously decide to breathe more quickly
when we run, to sweat when it is hot or to blink to protect
our eyes. We don't decide consciously to move in the night
during sleep to prevent our joints from locking and
becoming immobilized. We adapt automatically to all these
things.

But our conscious reaction to pain is different. An
immediate physical response is an increase in the physical
tension needed to escape from the danger we are in. If a
bull chases you you run like mad to get over the nearest
fence, or, if your hand is burning, you jerk it away from
the fire. But when pain is upon you, when you are burned
or gored, when the cause is established and, as far as
possible, controlled, the escape mechanism is no longer
appropriate. Increased tension only increases the intensity
of the pain.

Our reaction to pain is different from the automatic,
immediate reactions like sweating or blinking because it
is directed partly by thought and is affected by a variety
of preconceptions – what we think that pain is, how
important in relation to other things THIS particular pain
may be, what the expected outcome is; if pain heralds the

11

birth of a baby, that is good; if it is a warning of a terminal disease, that is bad. The framework in which we contain the whole pain experience determines the strength of tension we use to fight it, but pain is an inner, subjective experience. When we fight it we are really fighting ourselves or, like Don Quixote, tilting at windmills.

I do not suggest that the pain control methods I advocate should be used as an alternative to drug therapy. Often, they complement it. If drugs work without causing too many side-effects it makes no sense to refuse them. But, for preference, they should be used in times of great crisis only.

There is always a price to pay for help of this sort, as those unfortunates hooked on tranquillizers will agree. Emotional pain may go but the pleasures of life disappear as well. People who have been on tranquillizers for a long time describe the results as becoming like a zombie. The effects on adults are bad enough, but I wonder what the effect has been on the children of the millions of women throughout the world who have been under constant sedation from tranquillizers, incapable of any spontaneous emotional response to the needs of their children.

Yet there is a place for tranquillizers. Used in moderation, over a short period, they help in times of great distress.

In the hospices where I have worked it is the custom to give massive doses of morphine or diamorphine to terminal patients. As long as the patient was pain-free and content I would never question the wisdom of doing this. But sometimes these drugs, even when given at the highest rate, were still unable to control the patients' pain where my therapy, in combination with the drugs, would make them effective. I did not use the therapy without the drugs if the patient was already on a drug regime.

After major surgery patients recover much more quickly when pain is controlled. The quantity of analgesic drugs prescribed is limited by the fact that the patient is already saturated with the drugs given to anaesthetize him, so here I was given a fairly free hand and the results were good, as the nurses in the recovery ward will confirm. They asked me to teach them my techniques.

Anyone, whether they are suffering physically or mentally, or whether they are not – yet – suffering at all, can only benefit from learning to control his or her response to pain.

This book is divided into three sections. The first explains my interest and goes on to give some of the ideas, current and from history, about what pain is.

The second part describes the methods I have used on myself and which I teach to others to help in controlling pain. Although the methodology is simple it is not easy. It is always difficult to change the habits formed since childhood, and reacting to pain with fear and tension has become habitual. The chapter on heroes shows that this was not always so.

The best results I get are with patients who have a strong motivation to recover. They have sufficient drive and the courage to try a different approach. The reports from some who have tried and succeeded are then included.

The third section comes last because it leaves you free to take it or leave it. Many suffering people say at some stage, "Why has God done this to me?" It is an aspect of the consideration of pain which is either avoided altogether, by scientists – or made of sole importance, by religious. It is essential in pain relief to learn to accept it and to relax. This is not possible if, at heart, you think pain is an evil, totally unjust and destructive. Equally, an understanding of the philosophy or theology surrounding

13

pain and its problems does not, on its own and without methodology, help you to diminish it. Cardinal Veuillot, one-time Cardinal Archbishop of Paris, when he was dying and in great pain from cancer, said, ''Tell the priests not to preach about suffering. We don't know what we are talking about. When I think back now to all those wonderful sermons I preached about suffering!'' Sometimes even professional religious lose their faith when faced with the reality of pain.

The last section shows how, instead of wasting time blaming God or fate or bad luck we must take responsibility for our own destiny. It describes the visits I have made to Lourdes and how I want to work there with the ill and the handicapped for a longer term than the usual week-long pilgrimage, because the conditions there for bringing about a substantial improvement in both the physical and the mental condition seem ideal.

The purpose of religion is that it shows the way towards happiness and tranquillity, not by changing the world as it was created but by changing our human reaction to it. It is not the world which has gone wrong, it is we ourselves. Every religious tradition is based in disciplines which combine with the grace received from God in bringing us each day nearer to a state of peace, even when pain is at its most severe. By developing our powers of self-healing we come closer to understanding this. We come nearer to God.

PART ONE

1

Living and Partly Living

I am interested in pain, but the reason I have spent thirty years working around the subject is because I dislike it so much, and because I can never be sure of escaping it, no matter how hard I may try.

No one can avoid pain altogether; the Queen, the Pope, the President of the USA or of the USSR, none of them, with all their wealth and power, can ensure for themselves or for their children a life free from pain, whether it be physical or mental.

We may be sophisticated but we are still superstitious. We feel that if we do certain things, obey certain rituals, follow prescribed patterns of behaviour, we should, in justice, be protected from ill fortune. It is because we feel so helpless and have so little power to control pain that we become superstitious about it. We feel that as long as we are "good" (whatever that may mean), and obey the rules (and those we generally make up as we go along), we should be able to claim exemption. Pain should only happen to those who are bad, who won't obey anything. They are the ones who should suffer, become ill, fall prey to accidents. "Why", we say, "has this happened to me?"

We no longer put our faith in corn-dollies in the house or horseshoes above the door, because since the advent of psychology we are less simplistic. We blame ourselves when we suffer, for our lack of positive thinking, our tendency to be accident-prone or our subconscious motivation; we blame others for their insensitivity, clumsiness or deliberate malice; and most of all we blame God.

We cannot barter with our own future. We cannot expect repayment in kind for the efforts we make. Our future can neither be bought nor even predicted. The incidence of pain is neither fair nor just – it is not a punishment, it is an incident.

We may know this intellectually, but the emotions which form our opinions and generate the drive to action are rarely guided by the intellect. We only pretend that they are. Our opinions, particularly those which concern so emotive a subject as pain, are rooted in preconceptions and prejudice.

We cannot, no matter how we try, ensure that our lives will be pain-free. The events of the future, the whole pattern of cause and effect, is too vast and too complex to predict, let alone control. Pain comes unannounced, unexpectedly, and if we are not prepared, if we are not trained or have been wrongly trained in the way to react to it, it will overwhelm us like sea waves following a tornado.

My interest is in teaching myself and others how to cope with pain. I don't like it. I know I cannot buy immunity from it either with money or with influence. The next best thing is to learn how to deal with it, to grasp the nettle instead of running away. Then, and only then, is life free from fear.

As a child my first memory of physical pain was in going to the dentist at the age of eight. He was a tall, mild man called Mr Middleton, wearing a white coat and smelling, especially about the hands invading my mouth, of disinfectant.

The practice of dentistry in those days was primitive in comparison with what it is now. The drill was a rattling, vibrating, screaming monster. My mouth was prised open and fixed so that I could not swallow the saliva threatening

18

to drown me, and the pain from every tortured nerve-ending drove me near to hysteria.

I was the youngest of the local doctors' daughters. My father had fought with distinction in the First World War. His medals and citations for bravery were displayed on special occasions only, but their existence was a glittering backcloth to our standards of behaviour.

I felt I had to be brave too but I wasn't. I screamed, I cried, I roared. My mother, a doctor too, and Mr Middleton traversed every possible route to calm me, from encouragement and gentle exhortation through embarrassment and mild contempt to open anger. Nothing worked. An abscess was lanced, a tooth removed, the decaying holes filled but God knows how they did it.

I was a shattered wreck afterwards, sobbing and snorting and deeply, horribly ashamed. I had been overwhelmed, taken over by the pain until all self-control, all the pathetic scraps of dignity so precious to a child in the process of growing, were dispersed. I felt that I had been reduced from a potential something to a complete nothing.

I was, by nature, a happy, secure child but for the first time I knew real fear. This experience could well recur and I had learned nothing of any value from it. I knew no better afterwards how to handle pain than I had done at the time. So I was afraid.

Learning to control the senses is part of the process of growing up and achieving independence. It is essential to the natural optimism of childhood, but the natural response to acute pain, other than the desire to get away from it, is not a part of the learning process. The fear, the tension, the tears do not, like other experiments we make with the senses, teach us how to handle the situation better. They even make things worse. I turned away if I saw Mr Middleton in the street. I hoped I would never meet him again.

The next time I was defeated by pain was when I was fifteen and my father died. This was pain of a different category. Although it was emotional rather than physical its effects were surprisingly similar.

I was helpless, I couldn't control what had happened. I couldn't make him alive when he was dead. I hated and feared the irrevocability of it, as I think we all do.

One Christmas I had left a new doll propped up against a fireguard, and its head scorched and melted. It was not the doll I grieved for, as I hardly knew it. The sadness was in that I could not change what had happened.

> The Moving Finger writes; and, having writ,
> Moves on: nor all your Piety nor Wit
> Shall lure it back to cancel half a Line,
> Nor all your Tears wash out a Word of it.

Learning by change is the essential hope for a child. Just being a child is like having L-plates on – people are tolerant and forgiving. But death denies learning. There was nothing I could do to help my father. There was nothing he could do to help me.

Emotional pain made me ashamed too, because I could not control it in its acute phase. I could not stop crying when my uncle took me into a newspaper shop and the owner, a patient, asked how my father was. I knew that crying didn't help and was only an embarrassment to everyone but I couldn't stop.

This pain was made worse because I could see no end to it. I knew that at some stage Mr Middleton would either stop to have his tea or throttle me, but the loss of my father was timeless. I tried to orientate it in time by telling myself that after eighteen months I must feel better. Everyone said that time heals, so I only had to hold on for eighteen months or so and it would be over, but a lot can happen in eighteen months. It takes a very long time to pass.

The result of these and other encounters with pain was that I was diminished by it. It made me, for the first time, fearful. This type of fear is negative and narrowing. It serves no useful purpose. It is not always recognized by other people but it gnaws internally and life, which could be full and vibrant, becomes mousey and colourless.

Decisions are reached where the overriding factor becomes safety. The years ahead are planned to conform to a predictable pattern. The spark of the soul is muffled, hidden beneath layer upon layer of cottonwool security.

Fear is essentially looking ahead with dread, and the dread is of pain, the pain of sorrow or loss or of physical suffering.

Living with any sort of fear is not living – it is partly living. I can't remember ever making conscious long-term plans about the direction my life should take but, in retrospect, I see that I must have realized, subconsciously, how important it was for my survival to learn how to handle pain. I knew I couldn't avoid it. No one can.

When I was nineteen I gave up the study of music, which had been my main preoccupation from the age of six, and went to study with Gertrud Heller at Crichton Royal mental hospital in Dumfries. She was an ex-dancer teaching a unique form of relaxation therapy based on pain control. I was her pupil for some time and then took over a large part of the teaching.

Relaxation as a therapeutic concept was an unknown quantity in those days. Most people sniggered when they heard of it. There was much more conformity then to the accepted patterns of behaviour, which were of the "keep a stiff upper lip" variety. I remember Winston Churchill, when a friend of his, who was as mad as a hatter, was admitted to the hospital, sending her a copy of a book about the Charge of the Light Brigade to fortify her.

In normal society the tensions of the inside self were submerged but mental patients exhibited these tensions freely. If they wished to shout or roar or cry or laugh, they did so. If they did not want to wear clothes they took them off. Nonconformity was an illness which had to be hidden away, because society can only cope with minor eccentricities.

The tension of many of the patients was that of *ebullitio*, of boiling over, and it had to be controlled. The tensions in "normal" society were those of repression, of loss of spontaneity, of luke-warmness, and they often went unrecognized as painful conditions. Pain is relative. If you don't know joy you don't recognize its absence as being painful.

Now the pendulum has swung the other way, and it is normal to boil over, using drugs and loud, persistent hypnotic rhythms to induce a frenetic sense of pseudo-freedom.

Relaxation challenges conformity whichever way it may swing. One of the aims of the teaching is to recover spontaneity and to de-condition oneself from pre-conceptions. Learning to relax is pointless if the circumstances you are in have to be controlled first. Anyone can relax in a protected environment, with sweet music playing in a warm scented room that looks like Barbara Cartland's. But there is no guarantee that life will be pink, warm or scented. The real value of relaxation is when you can relax if the going is tough, when you are in danger or in pain.

It doesn't come naturally to relax at such times. Instinctively, when danger threatens, the eyes glaze, the body tightens, breathing becomes shallow and the mind freezes. Gertrud Heller put her students into stressful situations and then showed them how to cope.

This was what I wanted. I was a pianist and I went to her originally for help with playing in public. When I saw and understood the scope of the problems she was tackling a career in music, even though I wanted it and had trained for so long, paled into insignificance. I went to work with her as an apprentice and later became her assistant, running groups of patients as she did.

I worked at Crichton Royal for three years until I became restless. I wanted to see the world. When I asked Dr Mayer-Gross, the psychiatrist who was interested in my career, whether I should get some recognized qualifications at the university he said, "No. If you want to read books I will give you books, but if you want to learn about people and become a therapist work here in the hospital."

I saw as much suffering at the Crichton as I have ever seen since. I saw patients who mutilated themselves, slashing their faces and bodies. I saw catatonic schizophrenics stand motionless all day by the foot of the bed, with one leg twisted, rigid, around the other. I unlocked the door of a closed, chronic ward to be confronted by an elderly, white-haired woman standing perfectly still with a large knife clasped in her hand. The ward nurses laughed when I registered alarm. "She stands like that all day", they said.

The manic patients, thin and febrile, moved jerkily, frighteningly unaware of the people around them. The obsessional patients walked forwards and then back again to make sure they had "got it right", continually washing their hands like Lady Macbeth. They took hours to dress because it was so important to put each garment on the "right" way. But which was the right way?

Sometimes schizophrenics talked back to the voices they

heard. Sometimes they talked to God sitting on their shoulder. He rarely seemed to say pleasant things.

After I left the Crichton I worked in private practice with rooms in Wimpole Street, and I worked in a rehabilitation centre where my patients had physical, not mental, disabilities. I married and had four children. When they were old enough for school we moved to Oxford, where I was asked to teach at the Dominican Priory. This led to my giving courses at conference centres all over Britain and in Ireland.

When my husband died I went back to working in medicine at the local pain relief unit. The results were good and I was asked to work at Sir Michael Sobell House hospice. A report of the study I did there was published in *The Practitioner*, and as a result I went to work with breast cancer patients at the Royal Free Hospital in London. Since then I have been working on a research project in the Academic Department of surgery.

All that I have learned in theory about the control of pain I have confirmed through practical experience. I have had four children. I have had major surgery twice. I have had cancer, and I have been fairly battered emotionally as well. I doubt whether I would have survived had I not been taught how to cope with it all.

2

Over-riding Pain

In Sri Lanka certain villagers take part in an annual religious festival. Men, women and children participate. Up to twelve meat hooks are inserted through the skin of each one's back. The hooks are attached to pulleys, and the whole body is then lifted by the skin high up into the air, swinging from side to side.

The people don't bleed. The wounds do not become infected. They show no signs of pain.

This is not trickery. They are not given drugs or put into strange trance states. They appear to be perfectly relaxed and at ease.

They are all, young and old, able, consciously and deliberately, to over-ride pain, and the result is that they are relatively undamaged by a procedure which, if ever it were inflicted on a Westerner, would probably prove fatal.

If the mechanism for the internal control of pain exists, why have not we in the West been taught to activate it? Why, when we have tension headaches, do we reach straightaway for help from outside, for the aspirin bottle or for analgesics? Why, when they menstruate, do some women need pain-killers every month whereas others don't? Why, when the Sri Lankans are able to welcome pain, deliberately inflicting it upon themselves and smiling through it, do we spend so much time and money trying to avoid it?

The Sri Lankans have subjected themselves to stringent tests given by Western scientists. They are made in no way differently from us; they have no physical peculiarities; they don't function in any way differently; the only difference is in their relaxed attitude associated with their faith and their subsequent lack of fear.

No one knows what the mechanism of pain is, any more than we know the physiological and neurological processes brought into being by faith. It is relatively easy to trace the physiology of the senses. We can deduce how we see or hear or smell by working on cadavers, but dissecting a corpse does not help in tracing the pathways of pain. There is no obvious pain organ. There is no place which we can touch and say, "This is pain". That is why, in the medical textbooks, it has until fairly recently been dismissed as a puzzle or a problem or even a mystery.

Pain is subjective. It is an inner experience and it is invisible. It cannot be measured by anyone else, no matter how skilful he may be or how well equipped with technical expertise. You may be cared for by a doctor or a nurse, a priest, your mother or your wife/husband, but no one outside yourself can know the extent of your pain, and no one else, no matter how they may wish to, can suffer it for you.

It is difficult to explain to other people what pain is like because of the problem in measuring it. Virginia Woolf once complained that there are a choice of words in the English language to describe every other sensation except pain. It is a lonely experience and words are not much help.

Someone in pain may contort his face or arch his body like an Angle-poise lamp to communicate what it feels like, to make it in some way visible, but it does not help his pain when he does this, and may even make it worse. It serves only to show those people around him that he is suffering, and that he needs them to know. If they cannot help to relieve him, at least they must make no demands on him, for he can no longer function normally. On the other hand, the Sri Lankan hook-hangers, in harmony with those watching them, are not looking for help or relief and they show no visible signs of pain.

The whole concept of pain, how we understand it, what we should do about it, is usually open to misunderstanding. The sufferer must make those around him interpret his pain accurately, but there is always the possibility that he is deceiving himself or even deliberately deceiving them. We all know of the people who cry wolf, but we also know the dangers implicit for them when at last their symptoms may be real and they may be ignored.

Doctors must tread carefully when interpreting the pain signals given by their patients. It is sometimes fatally easy to match the pain to the apparent injury, saying mentally, "the pain should be this or that bad and, if it is worse, then he/she must be a hypochondriac. Send him/her to a psychiatrist." I have known several cancer patients who served time in a mental hospital, treated as neurotics, before the diagnosis was clarified, because neither the GP nor the psychiatrist could acknowledge the reality of the patients' pain.

This is not necessarily culpable. Doctors are not gods nor do they usually claim infallibility. The patient has to communicate adequately, just as the doctor has the responsibility to respond. Early symptoms of cancer are not always obvious and, if the patient has a history of neurosis and is unreliable in presenting his symptoms, the GP is more likely to misinterpret his complaints.

Interpersonal communication between doctor and patient is an art not a science. The signals picked up are too subtle to quantify, to generalize or to regulate. Every human being is unique.

Psychologists try to make communication into a scientific

technology. They try to manipulate patients by using pre-determined strategies of behaviour which will, they think, bring about a predictable response. If I say "this" the patient ought to say "that". If he is so ill-advised as to ask an awkward question for which there is no textbook answer, then the most effective strategy is to ask it back to him. The patient asks, "Am I very ill?" and the efficient counsellor counters with, "Do YOU think that you are very ill?" It becomes like Alice in Wonderland meeting the Queen. No one is any the wiser, but the psychologist has been let off the hook and can congratulate himself on having conducted a tidy interview where nothing got out of control, where no real communication took place and where the patient left as bewildered as when he came in.

Patients in a pain clinic sometimes ask, "Is my pain worse because the disease is spreading?" and it is very difficult to know how to answer. Protest groups are now insisting that patients should be told of all the possibilities and should have access to their notes. But although a doctor must, in private or with his colleagues, make some prediction as to the patient's prognosis his judgement may be completely wrong, and, if the patient is told that his condition is rapidly deteriorating then his pain will become worse and he will go down even more quickly. He will lose hope, the healing hope which generates energy, and sink into the despair which makes energy fade and dwindle away.

The doctor cannot know for sure what the progress of the disease may be. He can only give an educated guess, but that guess will inevitably influence the course of his patient's illness. This is why the patient would not benefit by having access to the doctor's unabridged speculations.

It is well known that we live up to the expectations we have or are given about ourselves. If a patient is told "you have about three months to live'' he is likely to die within that period, not necessarily because his physical condition has deteriorated but because he has programmed himself to do so.

A man and his wife, both patients of mine and both with different kinds of cancer, took it in turns to be admitted to a hospice. Their daughter's first pregnancy was fraught with danger and they felt that one of them must stay at home with her. They were both dying and so were admitted one at a time for pain control and rest, then they swopped over.

Their daughter's baby was safely born. The son-in-law came home from abroad to care for his wife and child, and both her parents died the day after seeing their grandchild for the first time.

When we expect pain we programme ourselves to feel it. No one knows exactly how this mechanism works, but it may have something to do with the incidence of phantom limb pain, another medical mystery in which an amputee often feels excruciating pain in a limb which is no longer there. He can see that his leg has gone but he still feels pain sensations. He doesn't want to, he is no hypochondriac, but it is as though his body has been programmed into pain and he cannot release himself from that pattern of expectation.

In the case of the hook-hangers they apparently react to other kinds of pain just as we would, with fear and tension, but the religious ritual programmes pain away from them.

Ritual reinforces belief. Doctors in the West realize the important part it plays in their patients' recovery, just as priests do. They dress for the part: a consultant wears a more impressive suit than his juniors, just as a bishop sports his purple. The consultant carries no bleeper so that he cannot be summoned. A bishop, too, is surrounded by acolytes who give and take his messages. On the ward the consultants wear white coats. They walk with an air of authority. At the altar the bishop sits in his own personalized chair. One eminent surgeon said to me, "We are all prima donnas". They HAVE to be, it is part of the mystique of the cure. The patient must believe in his doctor's omniscience or he would never submit himself for surgery. If he gave himself time to consider the grounds he has for allowing a perfect stranger to inject drugs into him, rendering him unconscious, and then to take a knife and cut into his body, removing from it whatever parts he so wishes, the patient might well, were he not overwhelmed by the ritual, refuse.

The ritual of the Grand Round in a teaching hospital is such that the patient is often intimidated. The whole hierarchy of medicals, from the professor down to the lowliest student, sweeps through the ward, stopping at every bed. The patient gets very little information from it, usually being too embarrassed and confused to ask the questions he has prepared. But it is great theatre, and afterwards he is left feeling how lucky he is to be the object of such distinguished attention. He feels confident. He feels better. His pain, with his anxiety, is eased.

No one specialty in medicine can claim to have the answer to pain, either in practical or in theoretical terms, but most patients when they see a specialist consultant do so because they are in pain and, although pain has been a problem since the world began, we still don't know exactly what it is.

Aristotle saw it as being one of the passions of the soul rather than one of the senses, an emotion at the opposite end of the scale to pleasure. Spinoza called it "a localized form of sorrow".

Both descriptions allow for the element of the unknown, recognizing the subjectivity of pain. With the growth of modern science attempts were made to be more specific and to find objective ways of defining it. The specificity theory embraced by Descartes suggests that there is a simple route whereby pain signals travel to the spinal cord and from there on up into the brain. There the message is decoded and orders are sent back to the body, determining an appropriate response.

This is partly but not wholly true. There are areas of the brain which govern specific reactions, but the understanding of modern neurology shows that the mechanism of pain is much more complex than the bell-rope reaction described by Descartes – when the rope is pulled on the ground the bell rings in the tower. It was even thought at one time that if the messages were re-routed to reach other parts of the brain we would be able to see thunder and hear lightning!

If it were that simple we would all react in the same way to specific injuries, and it would be possible to predict what the response would be from the extent and severity of the damage. This is not so. Patients coming out of the theatre after major surgery all react differently, even though the operation, the surgeon performing it, and the anaesthetist may all have been the same.

Another scientific attempt to define pain is the intensity theory. When normal sensory perception is intensified beyond a certain level it is recognized as being painful. Warmth is pleasant until it intensifies into heat. Massage is a pleasure while it is gentle, but hard rubbing bruises and hurts. Again, this is partly true. While we all perceive pain at a certain level – when heat reaches 44–45° we all recognize it as painful – but how much we can stand thereafter varies from person to person. This is known as the pain tolerance threshold.

An American doctor in Vietnam noticed that soldiers returning wounded from the front line made no demands for pain-killers, while his patients in the USA who had similar injuries inflicted by surgery needed strong opiates to dull the pain. He concluded that the soldiers were so relieved at getting away from the line of battle that their injuries were not a threat to them, they were almost a relief, whereas surgery was the worst experience of his patients in America. They were afraid and they felt pain. The soldiers were not afraid so they did not react with the tension which exacerbates pain.

Pain and fear are closely linked. Fear, anxiety, apprehension all manifest themselves in a state of physical tension. Once we know how to reduce that tension, we are on the way to controlling pain.

Contrary to many opinions, levels of pain tolerance are not genetically determined. If a mother screams with alarm every time her child falls and scrapes himself, the child is likely to take this reaction on board and to develop a low threshold of tolerance, being programmed by his mother to do so. But this is nurture not nature. With appropriate help and training we can all heighten the level of our tolerance, de-programme ourselves from fear, and ease our pain.

A theory was proposed some years ago when a psychologist and a physiologist combined to work on the mechanisms of pain. They suggested that cutaneous pain is transmitted along two sets of nerve fibres: short fibres transmit acute pain, long fibres transmit prolonged pain. The messages travelling along the nerves arrive at the dorsal horns of the spinal column where they are met by signals coming down from the brain; the eyes have seen the danger approaching, the gun in the raised hand, the fire coming too close, the fist ready to strike, and the brain sends down signals which may modify the pain response. It may be more practical in terms of survival to run like crazy rather than to bother about the pain and how badly one has been hurt. The brain makes this assessment and over-rides the pain signals. Similarly a footballer may play on because his desire to win over-rides the pain from a broken leg.

Playing tennis or golf after a long break exercises muscles unused to activity, and they react by emitting pain signals, but the brain has already worked out that there is no cause for alarm. Muscle stiffness, although extremely painful and sometimes almost paralysing in its effect, is not threatening, so it is not even called pain. It is called stiffness and people laugh rather than sympathize.

But if the sportsman were told that his symptoms were caused by some muscular wasting disease, he would respond to the pain very differently. He would be tense and afraid and become immobile to protect himself. He would call the pain "pain" and it would worsen.

We in the West have been trained and conditioned since childhood, firstly by our over-anxious mothers and then by the values of society, to be afraid of pain, to see it as an enemy to fight and to repel. Television advertisements don't say, "Relax and learn to ease it" when showing someone in pain. They say, "Take this pill or that pill and they will make you relaxed enough for your headache to go". They implant attitudes which make us think we have to buy our way out of pain. In subtle ways they tell us that we DESERVE relief from it; that it is one of our rights to lead a pain-free life.

Ridding the world completely from pain is not the answer, because pain is not an easy enemy. It can even, in rare cases, become a friend. A neuro-surgeon may be delighted when the child on which he has operated feels pain. It means that the nerves are still functioning and the operation has been a success.

Pain has an essential part to play in our survival, as it warns us of danger. You might suppose that anyone congenitally incapable of feeling pain is to be envied, but this is not so. Some people are born without the capacity to feel pain – they burn themselves without noticing, or they lie still through the night, with the result that their joints become deformed because they don't feel the pain which warns them to move. Children with this condition can poke out their own eyes or bite through their tongues while eating. There is even one story in the medical textbooks that reads like a sick joke from a silent movie: a bride cooking her husband's meal picks up the casserole dish with her bare hands and puts it on the hardboard table which immediately bursts into flames.

Another medical story describes a doctor who, because his daughter could feel no pain, sent her to his colleagues at the university for tests. She was placed in hot water and then freezing cold. She was subjected to electric shocks and punctured with needles. Whatever they did to her she showed no signs of pain, but she died at the age of twenty-nine from a massive infection which could not be controlled. Just before she died she complained of pain.

We learn through suffering pain. The Latin root of the verb "to learn" means "to suffer". When a new-born baby can't breathe the midwife slaps him to make him cry. Pain is the stimulus which gets his metabolism going. Learning is like a cautionary tale. There are myriads of options from which we can choose: a foot can be placed this way or that way; if we touch something soft it feels good, if we touch a razor it hurts. The choice is guided by pain.

We know as children how to over-ride pain. A child

recognizes when the function of pain is to teach, and he is not afraid. He hurts himself continually in learning how to adjust to the world around him, and to find order in the chaos of sensory impressions with which he is bombarded, but his crying is more from anger and frustration than from fear. He gets up when he falls and tries again in a different way. He uses pain. He tries to avoid it, but if he were in extreme fear he would give up any attempt to make progress, and to learn to adapt, he would remain quiet, still and tense, afraid to take any more chances.

By the time we reach adulthood the delight in learning which we all had as children, has usually either been lost, killed or buried. By then we have evolved paradigms of behaviour and belief which act as safeguards, replacing the actuality of sensory experience. We place our trust in prediction. We have programmed ourselves or been programmed into clinging to a pre-ordained set of values and ideas of what we are and what we should think. We don't often change. Education becomes a process of conditioning, and learning degenerates into accumulating information and storing it away in the various pigeonholes of the brain for future recall. If we are lucky we are reminded on occasion to "come back to your senses".

We can trust to our instinct for survival in avoiding immediate pain, we get out of the way when a bus looms – just as it is by instinct that we walk and talk and do all the other things necessary for survival. But the instinctive reaction when we are adult and pain is upon us is to become tense, to fight and to resist it. The fact that this is ineffective, even making the pain worse, may be proved again and again, but we still react in the same way. We don't learn.

We don't seem to learn much from emotional pain

either, though this occurs more frequently than physical pain. The best psychiatrist I know said to me that people always repeat their mistakes. He then went on to prove it by marrying for the third time. For the third time he married a patient of his. For the third time the marriage ended in divorce.

As children pain teaches us how to survive, to change, to live, but when we grow up it becomes an ogre, a warning only of death and decay.

Learning how to approach pain positively not only makes living, when pain strikes, less unpleasant, but learning from it expands our horizons. When we stop learning because we are afraid of being hurt, we become static, even stagnant.

The optimism of childhood comes through meeting new experiences, and learning, by risking the pain of making an error, how best to adapt to them. When that process stops, when the new experience is fitted into a jigsaw pattern of thought already constructed, then we experience boredom, depression, fear. We no longer adapt to the world. We expect the world to adapt to us. We don't learn to change any more. We stick to the safe, well-tried paths. Fear of pain, of being hurt, of suffering, destroys the excitement and blinds us to the novelty in our lives. We forget how to over-ride pain.

PART TWO

3

Method

Relaxation, Breath Control, Controlling Emotional Pain,
Posture, Concentration, Using Tapes

Mastering the art of pain control is more a process of minimizing pain until it eases and sometimes goes away altogether than of learning magic runes or strange practices in the hope of destroying it. It is based on common sense. You start by acknowledging the pain and accepting it, and then you hack away at it until it goes. Sometimes, if you get the preparation right, it never returns.

This method devolves around sensing the true balance in yourself between relaxation and tension. This is reached through effortless concentration, an easy focus of attention, which recognizes any imbalance and corrects it by easing the free flow of breathing.

Both body and mind are interdependent. You can't treat one without considering the results on the other. A wise psychiatrist considers the effect that symptoms such as malnutrition may have on his patient's mental state. A wise physician will recognize the effect that his patient's ability to handle mental stress will have on the course of his recovery, even when the sickness may be as physical in origin as a virus infection or a cancer. A wise priest will acknowledge that a tranquil spirit emerges from an unstressed body and a quiet mind.

Athletes consult psychologists to help them to reach the right mental attitude towards their training. If they cannot concentrate on the will to succeed they will not win, no matter how finely their body may be attuned. Chess champions, using a skill in which one would suppose the body to play only a small part, train by running or taking violent physical exercise. The brain will not function at its best without physical energy to regenerate it.

My teacher had been famous as a dancer in Germany before coming to England. When I knew her, she worked in a mental hospital, and she helped her mental patients by teaching them how to cope with physical tension and pain. Relaxed concentration is the key. Through it you begin to understand the way your body and mind influence each other. You do no good to either by trying to achieve control by force, by strained effort of the will, by added tension.

We, her students, learned how much physical or mental pain can be made worse by the way the patient reacted to it emotionally. It was then no great jump to understand that emotional suffering, too, can be controlled, that emotion is in part physical, and that physical pain is in part emotional. We realized that the extent of the patient's suffering was, to a degree, within his own control. The way in which he reacted to it either eased it or made it worse. Much of his suffering could be eased by himself, with no drugs or help from outsiders, once he had been taught what to do.

We were asked to lie on a hard wooden floor so that we could increase our awareness of the tension of our bodies – the first step in learning to relax. If you lie on a soft bed the bed relaxes all right, but not necessarily the body on it, which may well toss and turn all night, never finding ease.

This is the first challenge, the first step towards taking active control and grasping the nettle. You know very well that the floor won't change its texture, so you have to change your response to it. Instead of becoming more tense you must let go and relax. You change YOUR texture.

It is a new approach. Instead of comfort and solace, gentle nurses or healing prelates, cushions under the head and a kindly ear to listen, you are invited to confront your own discomfort and adjust to it, to help to heal yourself. If you can do this positively the long-lost optimism of childhood and the quest for independence return. Hope, one of the cardinal virtues, is renewed.

Psychologists and the lesser breeds they attach to themselves, counsellors and the like, often categorize their patients as though they were set in stone or pillars of salt. They programme them to expect the behaviour from themselves appropriate to their category or to the text book from which it derives. The implication is that we are irrevocably set and conditioned, that we do not have the capacity to change; like an arthritic joint we have lost flexibility and cannot adapt to the world or learn from it. We lose all hope.

If someone is told they have a depressive personality they will remain depressed. If someone is told they have a low threshold of pain they will feel justified, even that it is expected of them, in making a fuss. They become imprisoned within their own, unchanging self-image.

Some years ago experiments were conducted at a school where the teachers were told that their bright children were dull and that the dullards were bright. As a result the children lived up to their teacher's expectations; the bright children failed and the dullards succeeded.

My teacher rarely commented on our progress. She told us what to do, describing the problems, and watched us very carefully, because you can tell by observation how far a person is relaxed and when they are concentrated. We were never in competition with each other. Each one had to discover for himself, and often those who found it hardest in the beginning turned out the best in the end.

Lying on a hard wooden floor IS uncomfortable to begin with, for the tension in the spine arches it away from the floor, leaving pressure on the head, the shoulders and the coccyx. No concessions were made in the class. No pillows were allowed, unless someone had a real physical necessity, nor any twisting to find an easier position. Tension can be as elusive to catch as a will-o-the-wisp when the surface with which it is in contact is soft. You FEEL tense. You KNOW that tension is there but you can't grasp it. You don't know exactly where it is. It will remain out of reach and out of your control until it is pinned down and its whereabouts exactly identified through confrontation with a hard surface.

When you have found your tension you have three options open to you, the three choices available in any form of decision-making, whether concerned with trivialities or with epoch-making events.

The first option is to make an immediate change in the outside circumstances. Decide on a course of action and go for it, either by removing the problem or by removing yourself from it. In this instance the decision is about whether or not to lie on the floor, and the answer is a simple "yes" or "no". (In thirty years of teaching, the only people I remember refusing even to try were a covey of dignified reverend mothers who had brought their flock of novices to learn from me but said that they themselves would only sit and watch. In nearly every case, as the day progressed, curiosity overcame them and they slithered surreptitiously down onto the floor to join the others.)

The second option is the one we go for most of all. It is where we make the minimal positive decision, and it is the easiest because it requires the least expenditure of positive energy. We agree to lie down but when we get there we "endure". We don't refuse the invitation but we accept it grudgingly. We endure in an attitude of negative passivity. Essentially it is a state of waiting for some outside intervention which will make the decision for us. And it encompasses the "if only" syndrome – "if only" this were different or that were different everything would be all right. It is a drifting, a putting up with things, tense with frustration, until they are changed. The attitude is characterized by tension, and, just as, if you float on the water and hold your body in tightly you will become quickly over-tired and sink, so, when you endure in a state of tension, you cannot keep it up for long. That is why "enduring" pain with tension cannot last for long.

The third option is one of positive passivity characterized by an attitude of acceptance and by physical relaxation. There is a subtle difference between the concept of acceptance and the concept of resignation, with which it is often confused. Acceptance is becoming receptive to the real possibilities of any situation non-judgementally, knowing that things are in a constant state of flux, and allowing the response to them to be spontaneous, with no emotional anticipation. "It is", says Elisabeth Kubler-Ross, one of the pioneers in providing suitable care for the terminally ill, "a feeling of victory, a feeling of peace, of serenity, of submission to things we cannot change." Resignation or fatalism means opting out, not responding at all; allowing events to take over and to dominate us. This attitude becomes visible in the flaccidity of the body, and can be recognized and confirmed in discussion. "It is a feeling of defeat", says Kubler-Ross, "of bitterness, of 'what's the use? I'm tired of fighting.' "

Relaxation

At times it is assumed that relaxation is purely physical, that it comes naturally and that it is easy. This is not so. Often, too, relaxation or using energy in a way appropriate to the demand for it, is confused with lethargy. Our reaction against the reverence for stoicism and over-tension of some Victorian attitudes has gone too far in the opposite direction.

Learning to relax is a process of de-conditioning both your body and your mind; of freeing yourself from the tension of your expectations; of re-learning spontaneity. It is hard work. It is a process of self-discovery. It is simple but it is not easy.

The practice of relaxation is common sense. If a boxer walks forward into a punch he will be badly hurt, because the impact increases with the impetus of movement. But if he moves backwards, riding the punch, offering no resistance but travelling along a parallel route with it, there is no confrontation and the impact of the blow is diminished.

The same applies to pain. If you relax, offer no resistance, no fight, no confrontation, if you become a pacifist in your response to it, the impact of the pain is minimized.

The power of passivity is effective in world politics, as Mahatma Gandhi proved in India. It is just as powerful in controlling individual suffering. The maximum is equal to the minimum. What can be proven in great things can also be proven in the small ones.

The physiological mechanisms involved concern the production of endorphines, self-anaesthetizing hormones akin to morphine, freely produced when the body is relaxed but inhibited when it is tense.

A passive, relaxed response to danger or to pain does not come naturally. We become tense with fear, standing stiffly like a rabbit caught by a stoat or like a boxer with a death wish. The effect of pain is then increased and our own self-anaesthetizing powers diminished.

It is now more natural for us to be tense than relaxed. Tension has become so habitual in us over the years since carefree childhood that we don't even recognize it. To have an awareness of the tension which restricts you brings you well on the way towards the ability to release it.

It is when we can recognize and accept our tension that we become receptive to the idea of change; we begin to learn about ourselves, our resistance, our strength, our potential to overcome fear, and with it, the potential to channel energy into a concentrated focus of attention which can move mountains, let alone pain.

Acceptance IS relaxation.

I use the word "relaxation" with reluctance. Firstly it is ugly. Someone suggested that the reason for this is the intrusive "x", associated in the mind with words like "laxative". Secondly and more importantly, relaxation describes only a part of the process and so using the word could be misleading. I use it only because I can find no other alternative.

As with everything, the effects of relaxing are potentially either good or bad. Positive relaxation releases the controls imposed by the will which makes us hesitant and over-cautious, playing for safety and fearful of change because of the gamble involved. Yet the truth is that there IS no safety. We are in constant movement, in constant change whether we like it or not, and we cannot predict the future with any hope of accuracy. We do not even know for sure that the sun will rise tomorrow. We are gamblers by virtue of our humanity, and we are continually called upon to make our play. Our only choice is in the way we do it – either in fear and trembling or relaxed and with panache.

We have to make predictions in order to survive. We have to take thought for where we will find food or shelter, and plan ahead to establish patterns of procedure, but such plans can only be like blueprints. They have no relation to the reality which has not yet come. They must be flexible as the truth of the situation is seen to differ from the image which we have concocted.

Linking such plans with strong feelings is a total waste of energy. We say "I *must* get there in time", as though we had the power to whistle up the late bus or the delayed train and MAKE it chug around the corner. Allowing oneself to emote, to become tense, frustrated and angry because pre-conceived plans go agley wastes energy, our most precious commodity, and achieves nothing. If the world were structured differently, if we could control the complexity of the chain of cause and effect instead of it controlling us, we would be living in a world of magic. Instead of emoting with useless tension at the lateness of the train I would wave my magic wand and there it would be.

Relaxation is a means of controlling the inappropriate feelings which increase the level of inhibitory tension throughout the body. Fear and anger are the emotions associated most frequently with pain. When the body relaxes completely the mind automatically becomes tranquil and the body at ease. Frequently students say, "I can relax my body easily but I cannot relax my mind". This is not really so. Every thought and every feeling produces its own physical tension. The first priority in learning to relax is to become sensitive to these, often very subtle, tensions which can be maddeningly elusive.

There are as many different brands of relaxation

techniques as there are of washing powders. Some focus safely on the body. One of these, much in use in hospitals, suggests that the therapist should memorize a list of instructions to give to the body of the patient which appear to me to be way beyond the bounds of possibility let alone advisability. I quote from the handbook:

— Pull your shoulders towards your feet.
— Turn your hips outwards.
— Push your feet away from your face.
— Press your head into the pillow.
— Drag down your jaw.
— Pluck off your tongue and make it lie in the middle of your mouth.

All these orders are to be delivered in a loud tone, making no attempt to soothe by voice. Nor is the patient on any account to be touched. Such relaxation, which really seems a brand of stoicism, would appear to be a contradiction in terms, and would certainly be ineffective in pain relief.

At the opposite end of the scale is the relaxation required for so called "deep meditation", where the instructions vary from a straightforward command: "Do NOT get upset", to visualizing a lovely place where you are not.

Traditionally, useful relaxation techniques are innate in all the main religions, and sometimes, as in the East, they are explicit. In the West they are implicit in some of the disciplines but this is often unrecognized. They will be discussed in the last section of this book.

Learning to value tension is one of the important aspects of relaxation. Tension is not all negative, and relaxation is not in opposition to it as the good is to the bad. In over-riding pain we need to find the balance between the two.

If you are completely relaxed and completely without tension you are also completely dead – we have to tense muscles to move, to breathe, to think. Negative, unproductive tensions lie in the conflicts caused by doubt, fear, uncertainty. Then you get the push-me, pull-you syndrome, when doubt strangles energy, pulling it first one way and then the other. An enormous amount is wasted, until even the way in which we in the Western world move and walk reflects the hesitation and strangulated tension permeating our bodies.

We are members of the animal kingdom and we should say this with pride. Other animals – lions, tigers, dogs, cats – don't go to ballet classes to learn grace in movement, it is theirs by nature, by right. It is our birthright too. It is a delight to watch the spontaneity of a child's movement, but, as we get older pervasive doubt fragments any positive flow of energy, and we lose the spontaneous grace of movement so that it dwindles into a tense awkwardness. It is like trying to run a car while water drips into the petrol tank: it cannot run on full power, and every so often it grinds to a halt. If the body is functioning awkwardly to begin with and cannot move with ease, the difficulties of remaining mobile when it is in pain are greatly increased.

Either in movement or stillness a positive flow of energy directed by breathing helps to reduce pain. If you have never suffered acutely you may find this difficult to understand, but anyone who has had pain will know that instinctively you protect the painful area by keeping it still and tense, defending it from attack. Even the movement of breathing is not allowed near, and the pain is isolated by tension from the ebb and flow of energy travelling through your body. This intensifies pain. Protective tensions multiply, spreading outwards so that even though the injury may be in the stomach the hands become tense, the eyes glaze, the toes curl up. This tension serves no purpose and has no end product. It is only exhausting.

This is true not only of physical pain but of mental pain too. We use the same terms in describing both, and both respond to the same methods of control. If you are bereaved you FEEL the loss, you don't just think about it.

A woman who had studied this method with me sent me the following account of her experience.

My husband died suddenly and shockingly. After the first day, when I cried a lot, I was reasonably all right and did the things I knew I had to but, after a few days, I realized that every morning when I woke up I felt horrible. It was not the sickness of nausea but it was a sickness. Maybe it was what people mean when they say "sick with horror". I found that it became worse if I moved to a different place or woke up in a different room.

The horror-sickness, although it did not come from any disorder in my body, was a physical sensation. I knew that each morning I had to get through it and to get rid of it by letting go, by relaxing it away. Otherwise it might linger on through the day and destroy me.

It became like another job of work I had to do, a problem I had to solve. The moment I started to think of it as clearly as that I wasn't frightened of it any more – I didn't feel it was the beginning of my falling apart.

The worst sensations were in the middle of my body where breathing starts from and comes back to. It felt like jelly, jittery and uncertain.

When I breathed out deeply and relaxed the jittering subsided and I felt calmer.

Then I found that, although there was nothing wrong with my sight, I wasn't paying attention to what I saw, I was projecting my sadness onto everything and it all looked grey and depressing even though the sun was out.

When I relaxed my eyes so they widened and softened, I realized that the whole world wasn't broken up by my misery. The colours, the life, the good things going on around me – if I let them – could help and heal me.

After a while I found that I was better. I woke in the morning and the sickness had gone. I even forgot about it.

The old tradition of being allowed to mourn, to react strangely for a month or two, is right. Bereavement is a wound which needs time and work to heal.

When you relax and let tension go, firstly in the areas of the body which have tightened up in sympathy with the painful part, and eventually reaching the site of the injury, you break through the barriers of tension which isolate it. The pain, instead of being drawn up and ringed by tension, is dispersed throughout your body. The WHOLE of your body copes with it, not just one isolated part.

There has to be an element of forgiveness in this. When a part of the body stops functioning, is injured and in pain, we treat it as an enemy, a traitor to the whole. It is frightening so we imprison it behind a barrier of tension. Breathing – which brings life, sustenance and healing to every part of the body – is not allowed near to the injury.

When you relax you accept and forgive your treacherous body, as the prodigal son was forgiven, and you allow breathing past the protective barriers, You breathe INTO the pain and out again. The in-breath brings with it vital healing energy. Breathing out draws away the tension which blocks off the pain and prevents help from reaching it.

Your body knows a lot about healing itself if you will relax and let it get on with it. The function of any invasive treatment is only to help your body to help itself. Our animal nature, freed by relaxation, knows this. An Old English Sheepdog of mine was hit by a projectile sticking out from a passing train, which broke his pelvis and left him with an open wound in his side. My children and I took him to London, to the Royal Veterinary Hospital, to get the best advice possible.

The vet lifted him up so that he stood on his feet, and we were so shocked that we screamed. Blood was everywhere; the dog screamed too and collapsed onto the floor. The vet remained impassive. "If you can get him onto his feet within three days he will live", he said. "He needs you with him all the time to reassure him, because he is so badly afraid. Lie him on a mattress in the sitting room and stay with him. No vet can help him now. It's up to you. Either you are prepared to do it or not."

We sat with him all the time, taking shifts because it took two of us to lift him from one side to the other to prevent him getting bed sores. He lay quietly, peacefully and relaxed. On the third day he stood up and staggered to the door. It was like a miracle.

He lived for eight years, and could run and jump like any other dog. His back was X-rayed a year after the accident, and we could see clearly how the bones had knitted together to form a new hip joint where the original one had been shattered. I learned a great deal from that dog, and it influenced one of my sons in his decision to become a doctor.

In the context of pain control relaxation is not synonymous with lethargy. Being relaxed means using energy, sometimes dynamically, but without the stress of indecision – Will I? Won't I? Nor does it mean collapsing like an invertebrate.

When Sebastian Coe was interviewed after winning a particularly gruelling race the commentator asked how he managed the final sprint, where he accelerated past all the others to reach the winning post. He said, "I relaxed". The tension he was in was obvious to see. He was panting for breath, the struggle on his face was agonized, every muscle was strained to propel him forwards. Yet he said, "I relaxed".

That is not a contradiction in terms. He relaxed by letting go of the negative, conflicting tensions which impeded him. His desire to win was mitigated by doubt until he let that tension go.

That sort of doubt inhibits performance. It blocks the free flow of energy throughout the body, and the process of damming energy is potentially explosive. Just as water, when dammed, becomes either stagnant and poisonous or builds up to burst through the restricting banks and erupt uncontrollably, so it is with bodily tension.

When I worked teaching relaxation in a mental hospital I learned that mental illness is only an exaggeration of normality, it is like seeing our normal, hidden propensities blown up onto a big screen, distorted by size.

Obsessional neurosis exemplifies how the body's mechanism becomes blocked when doubt over-rules performance. I had a patient who spent so long dressing in the morning that eventually she could not dress herself at all. She picked up one item of clothing, started to put it on then took it off again. She could not decide which would be "right", to put her left arm in first or not, so she had to keep trying again. This went on all day. I taught her techniques of breathing and relaxation and then, to give her confidence, I taught her to ride a bicycle. Once she gave it the initial impetus and the wheels started to move at the top of a slope, she couldn't stop and change her mind, she had to let go. The people in the hospital thought at first that we were both crazy, but, after they saw her improvement and the courage and determination she was showing, they stopped to cheer her on. From being a candidate for a leucotomy operation she ended up working as an efficient secretary in the administrative department. I hope, if she reads this, that she is well and happy.

The world we live in is in continual movement like a kaleidoscope of ever changing colours. We can't stop the world and get off. There is no safety in stasis, as Emily learned when she rode her bicycle. Any movement, even breathing, requires both the contraction and the relaxation of muscles. The balance is where both respond efficiently and the energy to generate movement is nicely judged, neither too economical with energy nor too profligate. Rather like the wise virgins in the parable.

This only happens when the orders from the mind to the body are direct, positive and concentrated. If too much emphasis is placed on relaxation as against contraction the body is under-powered and insufficient energy is generated. This is what happens when we lose hope, when we become overwhelmed by fatalism and depressed. As we shall see later, depression plays a big part in the torment of chronic pain conditions.

There is a proper place for everything, and doubt has its positive aspects too. No one goes bald-headed into activity without considering all the options, but once your mind has been made up, doubt should be cast away. It must not overlap into the activity itself, for if it does it creates a negative, inhibiting, paralysing tension.

Relaxation is not only a peripheral skill which sometimes eases hypertension. It is rediscovering a balance inherent in all of us, between our own movement and the movement of the world around us. It is like swimming. No matter how scared you may be you have to let go of the side and kick off, moving through and with the changing patterns of the water. When you let go and trust the water to carry you, you can swim all right. It is in your nature to do so, just as it is in your nature to control pain.

Breath Control

Breathing IS life. In the West we take it for granted. We breathe with little awareness of what we are doing – either of what we do to breathing or of what it does to us.

Ordinarily we breathe approximately eighteen times each minute, 1,080 times in an hour and 25,290 times in a day. The purpose of breathing is to exchange oxygen for carbon dioxide. It is like the positive and negative current in electricity. Oxygen vitalizes the body, providing it with nutrients, carbon dioxide is the waste gas expelled as we breathe out.

The interest of Western doctors often stops with basic knowledge of this mechanism. When I told a consultant who asked me about the methods I used, that breathing was one of the most important aspects, he said, "Well, we all know what breathing does. Nothing." Doctors are trained to work on changing the body's chemistry by using invasive therapies, and they sometimes ignore the patient's latent ability to control his own chemistry.

There is a close link between the patterns of our breathing and our emotional state, and our emotional state has the greatest influence on our physical state. But it is not possible to control emotion through will-power alone. The outward signs of an emotion may be hidden by using the force of the will, by pretending so that the physical signs do not communicate to anyone else. But that does not control the surge of energy erupting in your body when a feeling such as anger takes you over. If you suppress the physical signs of an emotion you entrap energy which cannot then be expressed.

Relaxed breathing releases suppressed energy. By breathing out deeply and by letting go you come back to tranquillity again. In the East breathing techniques have been familiar for a very long time, both in the practice of religion and of medicine, as both search for means of relieving pain.

A Japanese psychologist, Takashi Nakamura, has produced interesting results from his work on breathing. He found, as I have done, that breathing-in deeply reflects a happy state of mind. Controlling and changing the pattern of emotion when it is unpleasant comes through regulating the pattern of expiration. It is an easy matter, through your own self-observation, to check these statements. Notice whether, when you are depressed, your breath out becomes exaggerated and you become easily tired.

When I worked in a mental hospital I noticed that patients who were clinically depressed breathed out too much. They lay on the floor relaxing, and sometimes I wondered when, if ever, they would breathe in again. Breathing out was like a sigh of despair, and the breath in was fragmentary. As a result, the oxygen intake was too limited and their metabolic rate slowed.

I tested myself and found that, if I was down-hearted and felt defeated, my rate of expiration greatly exceeded that of inspiration. It became a vicious circle. The more heavily I breathed out the more I became depressed. I found that taking violent physical exercise was the answer. Swimming, playing squash, running, all altered the pattern of breathing to increase oxygen intake and recover vitality. Then the depression lifted.

Depression is very often physiological in origin, caused by over-tiredness or a low metabolic rate.

I met a friend after a long absence and was shocked to see how ill he looked. He had been examined by one doctor after another, none of whom could find anything clinically wrong with him, but he felt lethargic and generally unwell. This condition had lasted for several months and he was deteriorating. I noticed that he was breathing out too deeply, and on enquiry, I found that he had been practising a brand of meditation which emphasized deep breathing and stillness. He had overdone it and deep-breathed himself into a state of malaise.

This is one of the dangers of practising meditation without direction, either from a book or under the guidance of someone insufficiently skilled. In one book on deep meditation, written by a Westerner, the group leader is told to encourage his group to practise breathing together while he gives them the beat, "Breathe out – out – pause – in". The author suggests that even if you have difficulty in breathing like this "you should persevere until it becomes your natural breathing in ordinary life". The ratio of breathing in to breathing out is one to three. I would hope that anyone practising such breathing in ordinary life had no strenuous work to do!

In the Eastern and Orthodox traditions great emphasis is put on the necessity for skilled direction while practising meditation or breathing techniques.

Relaxed breathing is a natural balance between inspiration and expiration. Nagashaki says, "Natural breathing is unconscious, untiring, easy, continuous and fine. It is neither long nor short. It should be smooth and well-balanced.''

Tension breaks the flow of the breath, but when you relax, *prana*, the vital energy sustaining us, is drawn in from the world around and circulated through the body, to every organ, to every muscle and to every cell. When you become sufficiently sensitive to the inner working of your body you feel this ebb and flow of energy rising and falling like a wave of the sea, reaching to every part of you, from the head to the feet.

The way to reduce pain is to relax, to focus your attention on the rhythm of breathing, and to send your breath through your body to the suffering part. As you breathe out the breath gathers with it both the pain and tension, and draws them away.

Yogis divide the ways of breathing into four categories:

1. **High breathing or collar-bone breathing.** In this the collar bone and shoulders are raised, the upper part of the chest and lungs alone are used, and the pattern of movement is jagged. "High breathing" they say, "is probably the worst form of breathing known to man, requiring the greatest expenditure of energy with the smallest amount of benefit." They list singers, lawyers, clergymen, doctors and many women among those who breathe in this way although "they should know better".

2. **Midbreathing.** Although better than high breathing this is still inadequate.

3. **Low or abdominal breathing** is of much greater benefit. The abdomen is pushed outwards during inspiration and contracted during expiration.

4. **Complete breathing** is "the king of them all". The

beneficial aspects of high, mid, and low breathing are conjoined, and the entire apparatus of breathing is brought into play.

Controlling Emotional Pain

On the whole we suffer more often from emotional than from physical pain. Each is contained within the other – emotional pain shows physical signs, physical pain is emotional too – but the origin is different. Emotional pain is not caused specifically by a physical injury. A friend passes by in the street without saying hullo – we tighten up in hurt. The family explodes in anger, as all families can do, perhaps because of something quite trivial, but we are left feeling pulverized. We are late; we are early; we are anxious; we are disappointed. We swing up and down like a yo-yo.

Many people can say quite truthfully, that they have never felt much physical pain, but the only ones who don't know emotional pain are those who have blocked themselves off from the impact of the world – the schizophrenics, the psychopaths.

Every emotional change is reflected in a change in the pattern of breathing, and it is through controlling that pattern that we can learn to control emotion. The disturbing emotions – anger, fear, anxiety – cause breathing to become shallow. The gentle emotions – love, kindliness – make breathing deepen and soften. If you can change your pattern of breathing you also change the pattern of emotion, you can change from anger and fear into peace.

The emotion associated most closely with pain is fear, and the breathing pattern demonstrates this. One of the clinical methods of measuring the extent of pain is by measuring the depth of breathing: if pain is acute the breathing becomes shallow.

There is a difference between controlling emotion in this way and repressing it. We have been trained to think that emotion *should* be repressed and controlled by the will. At school children are taught that they must not show anger or boredom or fear, but, as they are not shown any method by which they can change these feelings they can only either repress them or disobey. An effort of the will can only repress and disguise inappropriate feelings, it cannot change them. So the child at school pretends it isn't bored or angry or afraid. It represses any spontaneity of expression, showing only appropriate, acceptable reactions, until gradually it loses touch with the reality of its feelings altogether.

One of the reasons for the growing disillusion with religion is the gulf between theory and practice. A Christian is abjured to love his neighbour unselectively, even the person who may be persecuting him. Most Christians have given up even trying, reacting with surprise if they are asked whether they could love Hitler or a mass murderer. It is not because they don't want to put the tenets of Christianity into practice, it is because they do not know *how* to control emotion, and they realize the inadequacy of repression and pretence. (Christians are not asked to LIKE their neighbours, only to love them. Liking is a different thing altogether.)

Emotion, like pain, is difficult to define. It is not specifically a mental process nor is it wholly physical, it is a mixture of both. But an emotion is recognized by its physical sensation – we FEEL emotion, we don't THINK it. We know we are in pain because we FEEL that something unpleasant is happening. We recognize pain by our emotional response. We recognize the emotion by the surge of energy it generates, describing sensory patterns in our bodies. Although emotion involves the brain, may be stimulated by thought and can be brought under the direction of the conscious mind, it is recognized by the sensations of the body. We use the same word ''feel'' to describe both emotion and sensation.

In 1942 a study was made of a 56-year-old man whose throat had been scalded when he was a child, since when he had been fed by a tube going directly into the stomach. It was possible then to observe the changes taking place within the stomach when he was subjected to strong emotion. If he was afraid the colour of his stomach lining became pale and the rate of acid secretion fell sharply. When he was in the grip of long-term anxiety his stomach lining became red and engorged. The rate of acid secretion rose and eventually his stomach became ulcerated.

Health and happiness often go together, and the best thing anyone can do to help the sick is to make them happy.

The physical symptoms described by fighter pilots during the Second World War demonstrated the strength of their emotions.

— Pounding heart and rapid pulse.
— Tense muscles.
— Dryness of the mouth.
— Cold sweat.
— Butterflies in the stomach.
— Frequent urination.
— Trembling.
— Nausea.
— Wet or soiled pants.

All these symptoms were precipitated by fear. The men were in a dangerous situation but nothing had actually happened to hurt them; yet they reacted very physically.

Most of us know what it is like to be really scared. There is no way we can be reassured when we are afraid. Saying to yourself, "It won't happen to me" doesn't work, because we know very well that it — whatever it may be — COULD happen to me. None of us can control the future.

Pain is frightening. Yet the energy that fear generates can be positive. If you touch a hot stove adrenaline floods through you and you move very quickly away from it. That energy has been released constructively. But if you break your leg and feel pain, the fear which generates energy has no immediate direction. That fear is not immediate. It is one of the consequences of the injury. Fear of losing control, fear of becoming a cripple, of disintegration. Energy is bottled up, inducing a physical tension which exacerbates the pain. Pain worsens so fear worsens. Tension, the physical expression of fear, increases, so the pain-inhibiting secretions are blocked and the pain escalates. Then fear worsens again. It is a vicious circle which can be broken only by relaxing the cycle of tension or by some outside intervention, by invasive drug therapy or by diversion.

An easy test of how, by relaxing tension, you can change your emotional state, is when you clench your fists very tightly and hold them in tension. Notice how other parts of your body tighten up in sympathy. Notice the teeth gritting, the eyes hardening, the breathing becoming shallow. After a time you will feel the first stirrings of anger. Nothing outside has changed, no one has caused your anger. All that has happened is that your body has adopted one of the sensory patterns of anger and the emotion has been generated.

Then let the tension in your hands go and relax them, so that they lie softly with the palms upwards, and feel the vicious energy of anger subside. Feel your breathing becoming slower and deeper, the muscles round your eyes relax, your teeth come apart. The anger fades away.

I do not believe that anyone can quarrel while their hands are relaxed. The energy generated by anger floods automatically into the hands and they tighten.

Next time you are in pain let your hands relax, and breathe deeply.

Next time the family fights or the train is late take a little time to calm down. Don't waste energy worrying over the rights and wrongs of it all – the train *should* be on time, the family should *not* explode – you can't change what has already happened. Concern yourself, rather, with repairing the damage. Focus your attention on what is happening NOW, and let the surplus energy zizzing around in your body gradually fade away.

Posture

In learning to control pain, a training involving mind, body and spirit, the first, the most simple, the most obvious, the most undramatic yet the most important beginning, is to correct posture.

The design of our bodies is superb, but the conditions in which we expect them to function are ridiculous. We care for our cars knowing that if the balance of one part in relation to the other is out of true the drive will not be right, yet, when we sit, the breath, which is the body's equivalent to petrol and which has to travel from the lungs to the heart and right the way through the body, goes through so many unnecessary convolutions, requiring so much extra pumping energy, because we do not sit upright as we should.

Consider what must happen to the digestive system when we eat bent over like a banana. I have been told by a medical consultant that the banana syndrome is a contributory factor in many of the functional disorders from which an increasing number of us suffer.

In many ways Victorian children were less deprived than ours. For instance, they were made to sit up straight. Their bodies were erect and responsive, which helped them to remain alert mentally as well as physically.

It is like tuning a violin. If the string is too slack it cannot sound. If it is too taut it will snap. It must be at playing tension – and so must we.

We look for comfort by sprawling, neither lying nor sitting but half one and half the other. The head pokes forward like the top end of the banana, the back is curved outwards, compressing the abdomen and rib cage so that there is no possibility of breathing freely, no chance of digesting food easily, no possibility of generating the energy to respond adequately to the events of your life, particularly if the problem is one of pain.

Tackling pain requires all the energy you can summon. When you sit or stand, deliberately bending over like a banana, you become as soft and ineffectual as one. Vital energy, which is so attractive, so enlivening a quality in anyone you meet, is lacking.

Improving posture is simple yet fundamental to your well-being, to your health, to your appearance and to the effect you have on others.

The change comes from the base of the spine. If the angle of the sacrum is tilted inwards to allow for the curve of the spine above it, the weight of your body is in alignment, carried equally by the poise of each vertebra. If the sacrum is tilted even slightly backwards or overly forwards the whole carriage of the body, even the head, is out of true.

You can easily gauge this by carrying a book on your head – as the Victorians did when learning deportment, and as model girls do even now – and watching the change in the mirror. Don't let the book weigh down on you. Feel that your head carries the weight lightly, proudly, like African women who carry heavy burdens on their heads and whose posture and carriage is, as a result, superb.

When sitting, if you lean supported by the back of a chair, your spine is out of true no matter how upright the chair may be. The simple, positive solution is to develop the muscles in your back so that you don't need support, or to place a cushion between your waist and the chair, pushing your sacrum forwards.

Many of the patients attending pain clinics suffer from long-term back pain. Nearly ten per cent of those certified sick in this country have this condition. In 1982 33.3 million days of work were lost, and £193 million was paid out in sickness benefit, for those suffering from back-ache.

It is not surprising. Children are no longer encouraged to take exercise, and the banana syndrome induces a state of apathy. It is inflicted on our children from the day when they first go to school and sprawl on plastic, badly designed chairs. They cannot sit upright in them: the front part of the seat is often higher than the rear, and they are forced to sit with their backs curved outwards, their abdomen and rib cage squashed together so that their intake of oxygen is restricted. They cannot concentrate energetically when the position in which they are made to sit adopts the very same posture as that of a long-term depressive in a mental ward.

The body has its own wisdom. If ever it is allowed to, it will do whatever is best. It will adapt, as my Old English Sheepdog did, to changing circumstances, to disability, to pain. But we have to listen to it and interpret its needs.

Method

Most furniture is designed for lounging. The three-piece suites and the deep armchairs induce a curious state of tension – neither the body nor the mind is at rest, but neither are they alert. It is a position of great suggestibility in which you are at your most vulnerable, where both body and mind resemble the violin string which has gone too slack. It is a position in which we watch uncritically, in which we observe passively. It is when television exerts its greatest influence. Critical judgement, the judgement needed when controlling pain, requires energy. When sprawling half-conscious in an armchair this energy is not generated. Information from the television or from any other source, from a depressing friend or a worried member of the family, washes over the listener and is absorbed almost on a subliminal level. We are made defenceless, we easily lose hope.

I was asked to help an elderly man with terminal cancer, whose pain was causing him to lose mobility. I went to see him in his home. The sitting room in which he spent most of his time contained a giant sofa and three plush armchairs. They must have cost his loving family a fortune, but whoever designed them can never have had human beings in mind, but must have been thinking of the needs of an alien with elongated thigh and six-inch-long calf, with spine tilted backwards from the waist and neck permanently bent forwards. All the seats were only about eighteen inches from the floor, they were deep and wide, and the poor man lay almost horizontal. The effort of getting up was so great that he really needed a crane to help him. As a result, once he was sitting down he stayed there, bored, lonely, depressed and stiff.

Neither he, his family, the visiting nurses or the physiotherapist had adverted to the fact that he really needed a strong, high, upright chair from which he could move easily and in which his spine was erect and actively supported by his own muscles. If they are not kept in use muscles atrophy.

When we "come to our senses" we must include that which is the most important of all – common sense. This man was on expensive medication, his quality of life was diminishing as he lost his ability to move, his loving family suffered as they saw him suffer. Yet none of this was at the time necessary. Changing the furniture, using common sense, was all that was needed to lighten his life and to ease his pain.

Concentration

If complete breathing is the king of them all, so concentration is the culmination of all that is contained in the practice of relaxation.

> There is no doubt that the strengthening of all the forces of life is in their heightened concentration, and concentration signifies undoubtedly the basis of all progress. In love, in every passion which "works miracles", the psychic powers are concentrated . . . We have at our disposal so limited a measure of energy that the less we expend uselessly the more remains for intelligent application . . . The value of learning controlled quiescence cannot be doubted. (Count Keyserling)

I realized how immense is the pleasure of relaxed concentration. As a child I was a musician. In music, if your mind wanders even to the phrase or note immediately ahead of just that sound vibrating in the present air, you are not really hearing it. Your focus of attention is fragmented between the future, the past and the present.

When you let go of both the future and the past, holding on only to the present and hearing each sound spontaneously, you enter another dimension of consciousness, where both future and past merge and you encounter harmony. It is blissful. It is cheap, it is free, and everyone can do it. It is our birthright. It occludes pain.

While I was a child and played music I could reach this stage of intense concentration at will as long as I did not strain to do so. Whenever I tried too hard I began to doubt and I lost the power. But on the whole, concentration comes naturally to a child. If you watch children playing they are totally absorbed in what they are doing, and they learn at a much faster pace than adults.

In certain artistic disciplines children are trained to develop their powers of concentration, but the word is rarely used in progressive educational textbooks. It is no longer fashionable as an educational ideal, but it is thought to be of more value to allow the child's mind to roam freely, giving it no curb. He therefore never learns to harness his mental energy and his thought patterns do not achieve stability.

Television exacerbates this. Producers assume that their audiences are incapable of holding their minds still, so sequences jump from one point to another, using visual images as a stimulus rather than for their thoughtful content.

The word "concentration" has bad associations because it was used wrongly. My generation were forced to pay attention when our teachers shouted at us to concentrate. My music teacher, a lovely old character who, indoors or out, always sported a large hat covered with flowers, exploded with wrath and kicked me if she thought I was not attending sufficiently. Concentration meant trying hard, so I sat upright and froze in an effort to please her. I frowned and tightened up. It didn't work. I was not really concentrated at all: my mind was pre-occupied with the effort to concentrate, not with the music.

Concentration, to be effective, must be relaxed and effortless. Real concentration is when the whole of the mind is absorbed. It is a form of receptivity. Whatever has to be achieved, whether it is running a fast mile or playing the piano or just being happy and free from anxiety and pain, the whole mind is focused on IT rather than on ME achieving it. There is no room for the ego in real concentration.

In concentration your brain has to become still. When it is occupied with self-talk – even when it is saying to itself, "I must concentrate. I must exclude everything else from my mind because I have to pass my exam or win my race or control my pain" – it is fragmented, it is fussing. The talk is an irritant, like a mosquito buzzing around, occasionally alighting on something and then taking off again, but continually threatening and endlessly irritating. One part of the brain is watching, controlling, talking to the other, trying to energize by the force of will like a continual, internal tug of war.

It does not work . The energy dissipated in trying to force concentration defeats its own object. The mind must stop verbalizing.

The discipline of concentration lies in learning to withdraw energy from the area of the brain engaged in this incessant talk, the area which divides attention, from which self-doubt arises; and to focus that energy on to the object you have in view.

Concentration is the precursor to any high achievement. Relaxed concentration provides the energy link harmonizing body and mind. In the preparation for any sport you can see the participants withdraw from other people, gather themselves together, breaking off contact with anything outside themselves. They need solitude and freedom from distraction in order to focus their attention. If that concentration is broken they won't succeed, no matter how talented they may be or how hard they may have worked.

When attention is dispersed and concentration broken the body loses co-ordination, lapsing into disharmony. This can be seen in an increase in physical tension. When energy is concentrated it is like the free-flowing waters of a deep river bed, directed, controlled, reaching to the sea in strong, easy movement. When energy is fragmented it becomes like the waters of a shallow river, seeping into many different channels, wasting itself, losing itself, dispersing across the countryside with no direction, never reaching its destination.

When a person in pain concentrates and centres his focus of attention he conquers fear, which is, of its very nature, speculation about the future; and he becomes tranquil and calm. Immediately his physical tension is relieved and his pain is eased.

Using Tapes

I have made two tapes to help with relaxation. The first, *Relax to Concentrate*, was made at the request of the Financial Times-Waterlow Cassettes after I had done a series of broadcasts on the BBC "Thought for the Day" programme. Its aim was to help over-stressed businessmen, but since then (1978) it has reached way beyond the business field, and to people working in every sphere of life. *Woman* magazine has featured it twice in their journal, for the help of people in pain, but it helps both men and women.

I was very uncertain about the wisdom of making the tape but I have been proved wrong. Of its very nature a cassette tape is static. It says the same things at the same time, where the essence of teaching relaxation is in learning to be so perceptive of the student's needs and the direction he is going that you adjust and go along with him.

But on the positive side, the tape is very useful to practise with. It can be used at any hour of the night or day – pain does not occur only at social hours. I frequently see hospital patients in the evening, when their relatives have gone home and they are left alone and anxious. This is the time they need to relax and this is the time when the tape comes into its own.

The best way of using a tape is with headphones. It is private and the cassette blocks out any extraneous sounds which might otherwise be disturbing.

As well as *Relax to Concentrate* I use an assortment of tapes to provide diversion. Practising relaxation involves using energy to focus attention and, until this is habitual, it can be tiring. I gave a week's course to a group of very young nuns during their training and, after the second day, they were allowed an hour's extra rest in the morning because they were so tired. Relaxation makes you aware of the tiredness which is normally hidden. So, after a period of relaxation and when the pain is controlled, I produce a music tape or sometimes a story tape as a means of transferring attention to something else, rather than letting the mind revert back to the endless round of anxieties. This is most important.

One patient, a forty-year-old with terminal cancer, was so overwhelmed by the hopelessness of her deteriorating situation and so afraid that she might choke to death, that she drove herself into a state of panic where she could hardly breathe at all. She had to sit up all night, leaning forward and gasping.

She responded to relaxation straight away and lay back against the pillows, allowing her breathing to calm down. While I was there to tell her what to do she was all right, but, if I left, the panic took hold again. So I gave her the relaxation tape and I gave her a story tape to listen to, a very gentle story which took her into another world where no one was ill or talked of cancer. The two tapes combined very well.

I was asked to use this tape on a research project, to try to standardize the results for patients just recovering consciousness after major surgery. The timing was exactly the same for each patient, the same words were used, no one was affected by my personality other than as it came over on the tape. These were exactly the reasons why I did not want to use the tape. Using the tape is fine while you are *compos mentis*, but these patients were not. I needed major surgery myself around that time, and took the tape with me to prove how inappropriate it was to use in such a situation. I woke up in the recovery ward with an oxygen mask covering my face and a drip in my arm. A nurse covered my ears with the headphones and switched the tape on. I kept drifting away into sleep and back again. I felt drunk, saturated by the anaesthetic. I could not concentrate. I could not even keep awake. I listened to the tape but I kept missing vital bits as I fell asleep. Eventually I said to the nurse, "Will you take that bloody thing away". That was not the time to be using it.

When I worked in the recovery ward relaxation was successful, and subsequently I was asked to give talks about it in the School of Nursing. When I saw that a patient in recovery was asleep I stopped talking and kept quiet until

I could see from their expression that they were awake and tightening up, making the pain worse. Tapes cannot respond to that need, of course.

The second tape I made is called *Relax to Ease Pain*. I made it for a patient with cancer, an aggressive woman in her late thirties who fought not only her disease but everyone around as well. We first met in the clinic where she realized that her legs were paralysed. The consultant asked me to see her but she refused, saying that she had a meditation teacher already who would be able to teach her to relax.

I bowed out but kept in touch with her. When I saw her in the clinic, or when she was admitted to the ward, I talked to her and, as far as she would let me, was friendly. I thought the day might come when she would need me. Two years later she was admitted dying, her pain uncontrolled although she was on the maximum dosage of pain-relieving drugs. She asked if I would help her to control it. After the first session we had results: she lay back and the pain eased. It was then that I made a tape for her. She was a proud lady. Everyone knew that she had refused to see me, and I wanted her to have the tape so that she could use it whenever it was needed, but also so that she could practise in private. She was discharged, pain controlled, within a week, and as a result I made the pain tape, so that it would be available for others as well.

I still have reservations about tapes. They cannot be as effective as the real thing. But they are ideal for the purpose of practising, and until I have the facilities to train other teachers as I would wish, they are the best substitute.

*

For details of available tapes see p. 171.

4

An Antidote to Pain

From tomorrow on I shall be sad,
From tomorrow on,
Not today. Today I will be glad,
And every day, no matter how bitter it may be,
I shall say:
From tomorrow on I shall be sad,
Not today.

(written by an unknown child
in a Nazi death camp)

Pain is real. It is never my intention to deny the reality
or the horror of pain. Fairy stories may talk about the
magical release from bad situations, the happiness ever
after, the good being rewarded and the bad punished; holy
books may talk about the just God who chastises only the
wicked – but little children are still imprisoned for political
reasons or tortured and abused at home. Good, honest,
useful people still find their lives cut short by disease or
their security destroyed through no fault of their own.

The child in the death camp found an answer and, if
anything is proof of God's mercy, it is that there *is* an
answer and that it is available even to a suffering child –
the discovery that she could decide when to be sad or not.
There is an antidote to pain. Two patients of nine, Joan
and Richard, found the way to ease their pain. Here are
their stories.

I went to Joan's house twelve times. She lived on a small
bungaloid estate in the same village where she and her

husband worked as teachers. They were not the comfortable, old-fashioned country-school teachers you read about in lovely books like *Lark Rise to Candleford*. Both talked about ''rights'' and ''equalities'' and ''freedom'' so often that you could sense their insecurity, their inverted snobbishness and their resentment of the landed gentry or anyone better off than they were.

Theirs was one of the few houses among the clutter of bungalows, a modern three-up and elongated down, ''tastefully'' furnished. Joan's craft work decorated the walls of the sitting room. They were in their early forties and unhappily married. I heard only Joan's side of it but I knew, although she didn't, that he had asked for her committal to a mental hospital. The children, two of course, complained of the quality of her cooking.

She had carcinoma of the right breast which had metastasized into the bone. Her expectation of life was short.

When she opened the door I saw a short, mousy, colourless lady. She spoke in a flat, monotone voice but aggression emanated from her like seeping water. Her breathing was angular, shallow, quick. Her hands clasped and unclasped in constant agitation. Her shoulders were hunched and she walked with a pronounced limp. She looked a freak. If she had gone out and walked down the village street people might have stopped to look at her, they might even have laughed. But she never left the house.

She let me in and limped to the sofa. She said she felt safer if she lay down but she could not bear to be still. In a few moments she was on her feet again, shuffling up and down the room, dragging her leg, wringing her hands like Lady Macbeth. It was a constantly repeated cycle – the sofa, then up and down, up and down, then back to the sofa again.

74

Our conversation could have no continuity but from it I knew she was in despair and massively afraid. She was bitter and resentful about the hospital, and suspicious of the help offered. She seemed to hate her husband. She was worried about the future of her children, both of whom had behavioural problems. She complained of acute pain in her leg.

She had nice eyes which looked at me directly and, from the beginning, we got through to each other.

When I first meet a difficult patient I always check myself over to correct any fear I might, and usually do, have of failure. If I am ambitious to succeed my vision of the patient is clouded by concern for my own success. If I hope she will respond so that I can go home saying, "I won. I helped to make her better," there are two "I"'s to one "her" in that statement. My interest is in me not in her, and if that is so, I am neither seeing nor hearing what is really going on in her. I sense only myself and my own self-interest.

Egotism is one of the real dangers of being a quack. Orthodox medical training is so stringent, so disciplined, so totally exhausting that no medical student would have time or energy to indulge his ego, to become a "healer" specially sent from God. His colleagues would laugh him out of it and pull his feet down to the ground. Not so in alternative or complementary therapies, where "healers" abound, and spiritual directors sometimes accuse those in pain of weakness in order to set off their own strength. Without the supportive background of healthy criticism you have to watch carefully that the ego does not take over.

I explained to Joan how I hoped to help her. She was perceptive. She knew that there was nothing more she could expect from medical treatment, they had reached the end of that road. But she realized that learning to relax away the tension that was fuelling her pain, causing her almost comical rigidity, could only help her, and she decided it was worth a try.

I asked her to lie down quietly and, after she had jumped up and down a few times, I asked her why she did it. She said that by constantly moving she kept her mind off her ''terrible'' thoughts. She didn't say so directly but she knew that her husband was untrustworthy; she knew her children were selfish and disrespectful; she knew she was going to die, and to her, death meant annihilation. She was looking into a pit of despair, a pit of primitive horrors where fear led to a crescendo of panic which could only be suppressed by maintaining a rigid cover to batten it all down.

Joan lived, as most of us do, fulfilling the pattern of events anticipated for her by her parents. She had been programmed since early childhood to do so – as we all have. Their expectations for her were implanted since her birth, and she thought she would be happy when these expectations were fulfilled: she had a husband in one of the professions, a good home, and two healthy children. But the pattern had turned sour. She loathed her husband; she loved but at the same time disliked and was frightened for her children; neither her money nor her home gave her any pleasure because she had a terminal illness. She could no longer live in expectation of change, looking forward to the good times to come as most of us do. She knew she was going to die, and she had never even thought of that possibility before.

She did not try to pretend. She did not care that she looked strange and behaved oddly. Her life, which had been a carefully constructed jigsaw puzzle, had suddenly broken apart into disorientated pieces.

Although her main complaint was of the pain in her leg, and she certainly had cancer in the bone, I thought she might be using this – like the sofa and the walking up and down – to divert her attention from the reality of her situation. I wanted to being her back, literally, to her senses. Her mind was so taken over by horror of the future that she had lost contact with reality, with time present.

I made her close her eyes, although at first this frightened her: when she looked outwards she saw only fear, when she looked inwards she disintegrated. I wanted her to turn away from the outside and face the pain and panic which was wracking her body, to start reducing it by relaxing. I told her that the only quality she needed was courage, and this she had in abundance.

I asked her to lie as flat as she could without causing too great discomfort, and to keep her eyes closed. It is easier to focus attention and to sense your body when you are not distracted by vision. When your eyes are closed you can't see. The windows onto the world are shaded, so it is pointless energizing your eyes. They can rest, looking downwards into the darkness which is real. Any visual images flitting across your consciousness are now unreal, fantasy, like a child telling itself a story. Forget it. We are in the real world now. The world of the senses.

Go down through your body, not visualizing it, only sensing it by the touch, the contact with the floor and by its warmth. How, when you can't see, do you know that you have arms or a neck or shoulders but by feeling them from inside, subjectively. You don't have to convince yourself by saying, "Yes. I know I have two arms because all human beings have two arms and I am a human being". Focus your attention on your senses so that you KNOW that your arms are really there, or any other part of your body, by the life and warmth and vibrance within them.

I told Joan not to home in on the pain straight away but to focus on the parts of her body which had tightened up in sympathy with the pain – to go into the right arm and notice whether it was tighter than it need be. Each part of the body or the mind affects every other. Releasing the tension in the outlying parts of the body or the brain releases the tension surrounding the pain itself.

Focusing on the arm without visualizing it or thinking about it makes sensory perception more acute. The best way, then, to relax it is to lift the forearm so it stands on the elbow and then to let it fall. We are born, so they say, with only two natural fears; fear of falling and fear of loud noises. Letting an arm fall, even though it is known to be safe, engages the fear mechanism, and Joan could only let her arm down slowly, tentatively. She had forgotten what it felt like to be unafraid. I helped her by lifting her arm a few inches, taking its whole weight in my hands, persuading her to give up control and to let me take over. At last she did it, and all the weight of her arm rested in my hand. Then I let it fall.

Still she looked at me with distrust but her interest was now engaged. She found that she could only repeat the movement when she gave it her full attention, and that letting her arm fall was a pleasant sensation. The prison gates were, very slightly, opening, and the obsessive thoughts overwhelming her body and her mind were in retreat. Her mind could not be on two things at the same time.

When her right arm lay perfectly still, loose and calm, she felt the comparison with her left arm, still jerky with spasmodic movements. There is no such thing as replication – the left arm is not a clone of the right. Although we are inclined, once something has been achieved, to compare and direct from the head, trying to analyse and repeat the movement, this means that we lose contact with the senses. Joan had to sense through her body, making contact as she did so, checking that she was not visualizing, until she could feel the weight of her left arm and lift it spontaneously. Then, let it fall. The right and left sides of the body react very differently. Joan's left side was in pain, so she had lost confidence in it. Even though the pain was in her hip and leg, her arm was tense too, to the point of rigidity. We worked for a long time to release it.

By then she felt much easier, having realized that she was responsible for making her whole body suffer although the pain was only in her hip and leg. Once she could let her arms relax the tension in the rest of her body started to go and the pain diminished.

I led her attention back up into her head, letting her forehead smooth out, feeling the weight of her head supported by the floor, drawn down by gravity. She felt that her head was just another part of her body, on equal terms with her hands or feet – not Big Brother sitting up there knowing all there was to know and bossing the rest of her body about.

Then and only then I went to the most important thing: breathing. Trying to focus attention on breathing when the body is very tense only increases the perturbation. Drawing attention to breathing has to be slipped in surreptitiously at the beginning, but not until some degree of relaxation has already been achieved. I find it best to align it to the feeling of weight. As you breathe out your weight goes down to the floor, you let go control, and the tension flows out from your body. Then, after a slight pause, the breath in rebounds like a bouncing ball.

It is through the focus on breathing that a different concept of time emerges. Each breath is unique. It has never happened before and it will never happen in this way again. It is unique as each moment of a lifetime is unique.

Now is real; not next week or next day or even the next second.

In the transition from childhood, for protection from pain we have trained ourselves to rely on our ability to anticipate danger. We are always on the alert watching out for attack, either from people or things. As a result we spend our lives worrying, beleaguered by fears that intangible miseries might become real. Worry is as habit-forming as any drug: we cannot enjoy today because we are afraid of what might happen tomorrow; we cannot enjoy this moment of time embodied in the pattern of each breath for fear that the next moment might not be as good.

Concentrating on each breath as it ebbs and flows through your body brings a sense of comfort and peace. The movement is as basic, as essential, as the movement of the waves of the sea or of the wind. Energy builds up to a crescendo then overflows and withdraws back to the earth. It is as primitive as life itself, and Joan decided to value and enjoy the life she had left.

She learned to go into, to focus her attention, on her left leg, feeling its weight and warmth, accepting every sensation she felt even if it was painful. Each sensation forms part of a moving pattern, always changing like a kaleidoscope. If you decide that your pain is never going to change of its own accord you programme yourself into stasis, you inhibit change. When you relax you become FREE to change. You can start hoping again.

Breathing into the pain and then through it makes it disperse through your body. I talked continuously to Joan so that she could not easily escape, and gradually she did what I asked her to. After being with her for an hour she relaxed and lay still without moving. I left quickly, on a winning streak.

Next day I was delighted to find that she had been

practising. She lay quietly on her sofa and said that the pain in her leg had eased. Soon she was able to lie on the floor, forsaking the safety of her sofa. Her biggest task was to face and conquer fear, and this she did with a courage which I could only stand back and admire. We discussed fear itself as being the problem, not the things which were causing it. Fear was destroying her, not cancer.

Fears are like plants. Some are nutritious and beneficial, others are poison. When fear stimulates an immediate reaction the effects are positive – a bull charges; a bus looms; a fist threatens, and you react immediately, quick as a burst of flame, with healthy positive fear. Adrenaline is pumped through your system, stimulating swift avoiding action. Our ancestors had to move faster than their predators if they were to survive, and we have inherited this legacy.

We are no longer constantly on the watch for predators, but the primitive fear reaction survives. Our bodies respond with all the emergency alarm responses, even to imagined fears. We fight invisible enemies. Our bodies tense in readiness for an imagined attack, the blood pressure rises, the heart beat quickens, and then if we are lucky, when the danger is over we calm down.

The poisonous fear is slow-burning and consumes gradually; fear of poverty, fear of failure, fear of death, all of which are based on fear of the pain which might result. These are fears which don't spring from actual experience but from an abstract: its anticipation. This fear does not stem directly from the senses but from imagined, illusory sensory perception. It manifests itself in an unproductive, unhealthy physical tension, which clogs up spontaneity just as constipation clogs up the digestive system. Energy lies dormant, couched ready to promote activity, but no activity is appropriate because the situation is alive only in the imagination. It is unreal, a product of the mind bypassing the senses.

Joan was afraid both in the short term and the long term. She saw no future but in death, which was to her an unrelieved horror. She had no clear vision of purpose in life other than fulfilling what was expected of her. She had no belief system. Her life seemed not only brutish and short but like an accident on the face of the earth. Fear of the god Pan, the god of chaos and disorder, had taken her over, and she was in a state of panic. In the short term she was afraid of pain, of the debilitating progress of her disease, of the day-to-day incidents with which she could no longer cope – when her children quarrelled, when her husband went away, when she couldn't decide what to cook. She had withdrawn from everyone around her. She could no longer, if ever she had been able to, relate spontaneously to her family.

From the furnishings of her house and the delicate way in which they had been chosen I saw that she was a visual person, but now her eyes and her sight were clouded by despair, projected, like the monotone voice, on to the world around her.

It was not easy, but I taught her to relax the muscles around her eyes, to let them widen, becoming receptive to what they saw instead of projecting her own misery outwards. I told her to look at colour, to see and sense the delight of gentle blue or rose or violet. Under her drab exterior her underclothes were a bright, ghastly, shocking red, like the colour of pain itself.

Joan understood what I was saying quickly, and she was able to use seeing to become more objective and to break out from the prison of agony in which she was contained. She realized that she was projecting her despair onto whatever she saw, and she learned to reverse this, to become receptive, to respond and be soothed by vision coming to her from the world outside.

Her movement in walking was so strange and unco-ordinated that we had to work on that next. She said she used to love to dance, which inferred that at some stage her co-ordination had been good. I brought a tennis ball and threw it for her to catch. At first she was so tense that she dropped it, but after a while she relaxed her hands and her eyes, and she began to play and to laugh. Immediately her co-ordination improved and her natural spontaneous grace broke through. The stiff, wary, clumsy response was gone; she forgot the pain in her leg and moved freely and openly.

Once she remembered what freedom from fear felt like she could recognize the tension of fear as it built up in her, and release it by breathing out freely and gently.

Several problems occurred during the time I saw her, and I was glad, because we could discuss them together and devise ways of overcoming them. I gave her a visual analogue scale to complete each week – a line marked with "very severe" at one end and "no pain" at the other – and she had to indicate where to put the measure of the amount of pain she was suffering.

Each day her pain decreased until, in the fourth week, her sister came to visit her, and criticized her sharply, cruelly. Joan was very distressed. She could not sleep and the pain curve on the analogue scale soared right up. Once again, I was pleased. Here was the proof I needed to convince Joan that her level of pain fluctuated not only with the progress of the disease but also when she was emotionally disturbed. It was a revelation to her.

Soon afterwards her husband wrote a letter of complaint to the hospital, demanding her re-admission. At my request a Macmillan nursing sister was sent out to assess Joan's condition, but, by then, she had recovered sufficiently to return to her full-time teaching job, and her husband's view was discredited.

We were both busy and I did not see Joan for some time, until one day, as I was working in the hospital, I saw a pretty, lively, blonde-haired lady talking to one of the nurses. I didn't recognize her as Joan. Her doctor told me afterwards that he had never before seen such a radical change in a patient.

That was in fact the last time I saw her. I left the hospital but eighteen months later heard that Joan had had a recurrence. I asked if I could see her, but as I was no longer employed to work at the hospital this could not be allowed. Joan regressed right back to her previous state and she died.

*

Richard's story is happier and very different. He was a businessman, well-educated and cultured, but he still had something in common with countrymen in that he was boot-faced, monosyllabic. I could imagine him patting a favourite cow protectively and daring anyone else to touch it. He was a sceptic of sceptics. And macho. Before his illness he had led a highly active life, both in his job and in his leisure time. Aggressive masculinity oozed from every pore.

His orthopaedic surgeon asked me to see him after an epidural block, to ease his chronic, but mild, backache, had been followed by a massive viral infection. He had been in agonizing pain for ten weeks and had lost a stone and a half in weight. My visit was a last-ditch stand, an alternative to further investigative surgery.

His pain was so acute that he could not stand, and could

only sit up with great difficulty. It was the first time in his life that he faced the prospect of defeat. A man of intense pride and physical strength, he was terrified of losing his independence. He was afraid that he would never walk again, and that he could no longer face the agony he had been suffering during the past weeks.

He did not pretend to be anything but sceptical, and only agreed to see me because his surgeon urged him to. He explained about his back and the history of the past ten weeks, just as the farmer would describe the illness of his cow, and he looked at me with the same lowering eyes.

I explained very briefly how tension exacerbates pain where relaxation eases it, and before he could start to argue, asked him to close his eyes and to lie flat on his back. I took him through the process of relaxing, becoming still, breathing, concentrating, and could tell the progress he made by watching him let his arm fall spontaneously. Boot-faced he might be, but he was trying hard. I told him to breathe through the pain in his back and to let it relax.

Relaxing was a new experience for him. All his achievements had been won through trying hard, using will-power and derring-do. The power achieved through letting go was unknown to him.

When breathing out is relaxed, energy is returned to the centre, the power house, the diaphragm. Relaxing in stillness, lying flat and quietly, is like recharging a battery. Energy is drawn back from the periphery, the hands and arms, the eyes, the forehead, the feet and legs, converging on the centre. From here breathing in generates energy which can be directed to wherever it is needed throughout the body. Breathing out draws it back to the centre again. As energy is withdrawn from the hands or the eyes tension too is drained away and they are left soft and relaxed. It is a lovely feeling and automatically the pain becomes easier.

Richard was still suspicious but, almost against his will, he did admit to feeling better.

When I saw him the next day he gave me a run-down on his progress before I could say anything: how many times he had practised, the difficulties he had encountered; but he had slept significantly better.

I made him relax in stillness first so that he had a baseline of calm and respite from pain, then I started him on movement. He was all right now when he was still, but when he sat up his muscles went into spasm and he had to lie down before he fell. He was deeply afraid and his eyes showed it, for his body had never let him down like this before. He had been able to do more than most men yet now he was as helpless as a baby. He couldn't even urinate without calling for a nurse's help.

I taught him to take the movement in stages, instead of battering at it like a bull at a gate. First he must relax in stillness so that he could conquer the tension of anticipatory fear. Then, as he breathed in deeply, he turned on to his side, and then rested again and checked his state of tension. Using breathing again to generate energy and lift him, he swung his legs over the side of the bed and pushed himself up. He relaxed before his muscles could go into spasm, and, although he was shaking, he stayed erect for several minutes. Then I helped him to lower himself down again.

This was a big achievement but he complained that he still felt very weak and his back hurt when he sat up. I said "What do you expect? You have been lying flat for ten weeks. Your muscles have been inactive during all that time. Now you expect them to work straight away again. Give them time to gain strength."

He worked very hard after that, whether I was there or not, until he could sit on his own without trouble. Next he had to stand, and again we tackled it in stages. He sat on the bed, made sure he was relaxed and then, breathing in deeply to give himself lift and energy, he got to his feet. Immediately he went into spasm. I grabbed hold of him saying, ''Breathe out. Now. Let go. Breathe out'', and his muscles relaxed before spiralling out of control.

This was the breakthrough. Richard told me how scared he was, how never in his life had he imagined suffering such awful pain. At one time, early on in his illness, all he could do was to stare at a spot on the ceiling, trying to hypnotize himself into easing the agony. He had lost all confidence in his body, enclosing it in a protective barrier of tension. As a result, like Joan, he had lost all sense of co-ordination, and what should have been a smooth, easy movement, with one set of muscles taking over from another, had become rigid and jerky. By focusing on relaxed breathing his muscles were left free to get on with their job, and he could control the tendency to go into spasm by relaxing and breathing out.

We had been working together for about four days by then, and we were virtually home and dry. All he needed was to gain confidence and strength. He was very highly motivated to succeed. By the seventh day he was able to walk up four flights of stairs.

It wasn't all plain sailing. One morning he told me that the previous day he had walked too far, and only realized it when he was stranded four floors away from his room. He was tired and shaky, his back went into spasm and he started to fall. He panicked, trying to remember what I had told him to do – breathe out, come back to your senses, relax – and he called my name, trying to force himself to remember. He straightened himself up, breathed deeply, controlled the panic and he was all right.

By then he was wholehearted in his approval of what I had taught him, telling both the doctors and the nurses in his excitement. On the eighth day he returned home with all threat of further surgery, or any other treatment, gone. I never heard from him again, and although he affirmed that his whole attitude to life had changed and that, even in his work, he would be a different person, I suspect that, when the danger was gone, he reverted back to the proud, invulnerable man he had been before. Nine months later he was fit to play sport again.

5

Chronic Pain

When pain is persistent, long-term, chronic, your whole life style changes and you have to change too. There are only two choices. Either you do nothing, you let IT change YOU and you have no control over what you may become as a result. Or you work at it, learning how to adapt intelligently to the new situation.

You are not the only person involved. The change in your life style is as much a concern for your family as it is for you. Talk to them about it and about the best policies to adopt as a family.

We have survived as humans because we have had the power to adapt, but then we became too clever and we learned to make the world adapt to us. I remember the time when, if you felt cold, you jumped up and down to keep warm or you went, God forbid, for a "brisk walk".

Marriage was for good and all then, and, if you didn't like it, you learned to put up with it, until, often, it became better. If we ever dared to say we felt bored we were given hard labour to put us right, not entertainment.

Now the world adapts to us not we to it. Central heating adjusts the outside temperature so that the body has no need to change. Divorce is freely available for any time you want to change a spouse. Television, not religion, is the "opium of the people".

Change is the most difficult thing required of any of us. We will happily require a change in somebody or something else, but rarely in ourselves. This is why persistent pain can be so devastating. It can inflict change, unwanted change, on to a happy situation and destroy it, and often we feel powerless to adapt. We don't know how.

I have talked already about the personal fight against pain, about how, by accepting, relaxing, concentrating, the sensations are minimized. But you can't keep that up for ever. After an hour of deep concentration you need a break.

Then you must use diversion. Once the pain is more or less under control discipline yourself to keep your mind away from it. If the pain has been very bad and you are not mobile, use a personal cassette player with a good set of earphones, and play music to yourself or listen to a story tape. Don't let your mind wander back to speculation about the dismal future or regret for the carefree past.

But remember about staying relaxed: then the pain will remain at bay. Don't let tension creep back in without your noticing.

If you are mobile you must work at maintaining and improving this state. Again it comes back to tension. Keep the pain in its own place. Don't let sympathetic tension snake through your body. If you are walking, enjoy the movement of your feet on the floor and the sway of your limbs.

Remember that you can only register a limited number of sensations at the same time. If you can only recognize the bad ones you will become overwhelmed by the pain. Yet there are parts of your body which don't hurt at all. Look for them and be grateful for them. If they are not painful then, when you relax, they will feel actively good and you can replace the pain sensations with pleasant ones from different places in your body, maybe your arms or your legs or your hands feeling soft and warm.

Don't become obsessed by the pain. Don't let it take pride of place over every other sensation you may feel, for if you do, it will defeat you. It is just one among millions of sensations you could be feeling.

Sort out what the problems are. Persistent pain is tiring, depressing and frightening. It turns your focus of attention away from outside stimuli. Your interest, whether you like it or not, is drawn back to the sensations of your own body, which is boring for you, and eventually, boring for everyone else.

It is depressing because you seem caught in a downward spiral from which there is no escape. However this is not so. The spiral is largely caused by the tiredness, the depression and the fear. It is like seeing a boxer caught on the run, panicked by the flurry of punches he is getting. If he has a lucky break, the bell sounds for the end of the round and he can sit down in his corner and re-think, he can change; he can come back into the attack and win. His victory is not just over his opponent – he has also conquered his own tiredness, depression and fear.

I have talked about how, through relaxed concentration, you can change any emotion. You don't have to be depressed or frightened if you don't want to be. Consider the child in the Nazi camp and how she kept sadness at bay. When you are depressed your mind dwells on the future with dread, on the past with regret. Nothing in the world seems capable of bringing relief. Come back, away from the future and into the present, into contact with each breath you take. It isn't the things you do with your life that really matter – it is just being alive. Things may look very bad, but see how much of that misery is really fear of the future; how much is resentment that you may not be able to fulfil your expectations of life. The mistake is in having expectations. We know we cannot control the future – that only happens in fairy stories. Think of history, of the people born to wealth who became paupers:

St Francis, the last Tsar of Russia, the millions of German Jews during the War.

Remember half the pleasure of living is that it IS unpredictable. It IS a continual gamble. It can get unpredictably worse, but it can also, if you keep your cool and your mind open to it, become unpredictably better.

Depression imprisons you in a static misery, where the movement and change and vitality in the world seem to pass you by. Relax. Feel the world moving and yourself with it. Come back into the present and you will be all right. Breathe in and out smoothly, equably, and your energy level will be raised. Accept that things are different. Things are not the same for you as when you were well, but nothing, nothing, nothing is all bad unless you make it so. There are always compensations which you can work on – maybe now you have more time to spend with your children? You can teach them or learn new things with them.

If you are alone don't regret it, and above all, don't feel sorry for yourself. That is the real killer. Once you let self-pity creep in you are on a downward path, so don't waste your time with it. You have only one life to live. It's a game, but you can't decide for yourself what cards you are going to be dealt. You accept what you get and then play the game. Adapt and make the cards work *for* you, not against you.

Whether you are alone or not you feel isolated when you have chronic pain. No one else can feel your pain for you, and you know it. Nothing is more irritating than being told by some well-meaning person, "I know exactly how you feel", because there is no way that such a statement can be true. Pain is a subjective experience, and the experiences of the inner self are not available to outsiders, no matter how beloved they may be.

You can describe thoughts or feelings to others and they may be modified by argument or sympathy, but pain sensations are yours alone, and the only help outsiders can give is either medication or help in relaxing. Happiness can be shared and radiates outwards. Pain isolates you like a small death until you relax and accept it.

You have to be tough with yourself when your pain is persistent. It is wise to ration your expectation of expressions of sympathy, because it isolates you if you are continually the object of pity, and it puts you down. You are denied the opportunity to contribute. The way you can contribute may be different from what it was before, but the possibility is there nevertheless.

You may find that people around you can be sympathetic in the short term but not day after day after day. It is sometimes far easier for them to help actively, to lift or carry or to drive, than to express sympathy.

Sometimes when you feel sorry for yourself – and we all do, even when we don't have the excuse of pain – make fun of it. Talk about the ''poor me'' syndrome, and laugh at yourself as though you were an outsider watching yourself behaving strangely.

You have to be tough about medication too. More medication does not necessarily tally with less pain, and every drug exacts its price. Some cause depression or constipation, or can damage your liver or kidneys in the long term. And, the more drugs you take, the more you need. It becomes a spiral which can easily get out of control.

We held case conferences in the hospice, where each person was discussed and treatments reviewed. Sometimes all medication was stopped completely, so that the patient's system had a rest from it. After a short time it was re-started and much less medication was needed then to be effective. By the way, it is important that such stopping and starting should only be done on medical advice.

But drugs, used wisely, are invaluable, and it is unintelligent, even arrogant, to deny their help. When pain drags on and on it is essential to get a break from it if you can, although you must use that break wisely too. Notice how the moment you think, "It's four hours since I had my last pill. I'll be getting the pain again soon", you tense up, waiting for the pain to start, and, before you know where you are, there it is. Remember that your expectation of pain has a lot to do with its recurrence. When you catch yourself thinking, "I wonder when the pain is going to come back?", relax, focus on the sensations you are actually feeling, and keep your mind free from fear, from anticipation. Focus on each breath as it rises in your body, and relax as your weight goes down and you breathe out.

When you win, when you stop the pain from occurring, don't convince yourself that this was just accidental. If you really think so then try it again and again, until you prove to yourself that you can contribute to the control of your own pain.

However, don't expect miracles. Nothing is going to happen unless you put in the work to make it do so. But if you can alter your state of pain by even the smallest fraction, then you have something to work on, something to build up on – you have already won.

6

Where Have
All the Heroes Gone?

We used to recognize, admire, follow the lead of our heroes. They were, we thought, brave and unafraid. They could withstand the pains which defeated ordinary mortals. They were larger than life. They were people whose determination and confidence were so great that nothing could swerve them, not death, nor even the pains of torture.

The most outstanding quality of any leader must be courage, which is at the base of every virtue. Mistakes, misjudgement we will forgive, but cowardice in a leader is intolerable. Kings and great leaders were expected to be brave, for if they were not, how could they expect ordinary folk to follow and obey them?

At one time leaders had to win their position by excelling. They had to defeat any other contenders in contests of strength and skill. Then leadership became hereditary, and children were trained from birth for the position they would hold as adults. The belief arose that both nature – in the genes inherited from his parents – and nurture – in the education and training he was given – contributed in making the child of a leader a hero too and the best person to follow in his footsteps. It is a practical system, preventing the dangers and uncertainty of fighting for leadership.

Finding the Dalai Lama who, before the Chinese invasion, was both the religious and the temporal head in Tibet, embodies the two concepts that the necessary qualities are contained both in the nature and the nurture of a child. The Dalai Lama does not marry, so he has no eligible children to follow him. But his successor is believed to be a re-incarnation of his spirit born into the body of a male child, and the whereabouts of this child are unknown. When the Dalai Lama dies, a council of monks takes on the leadership of the country until they are guided into finding the new incarnation. They tell by dreams and signs in which geographical area to look, and they identify the boy by his bearing, and by his recognition of the belongings of his predecessor. With his parents, he is then taken to Lhasa, where he is trained from then on for the job he has to do.

The present Dalai Lama, also discovered in this way, proves the success of the system. He has the respect not only of his own people but, from the time when he was thrust on to the world stage as a political leader exiled from his own country, he has won the respect and admiration of millions of us in the West. His integrity, his honesty in a world of corruption, cannot be doubted. A coward has neither integrity nor honesty. The Dalai Lama is a brave man, and no matter how bad the present plight of the Tibetan nation may be, we can only envy them their leader.

Neither re-incarnation nor the recognition of signs and portents are concepts with which we in the West are familiar. I neither believe nor disbelieve, but I do respect the Tibetans' belief.

Both nature and nurture were relevant in choosing leaders in the West until the monarchies were stripped of their power. There are risks in relying on hereditary leadership. The child who is immediate successor – trained to be brave, to be honest, to be compassionate – may die, and the next in line may have had a very different training. Would Princess Margaret, one wonders, have made as selfless, wise and dedicated a leader as our present Queen? If her father had been known as the future king when he was a child, would he not have been better prepared for his reign and suffered less as a result?

Now we do not expect physical courage of our leaders, who are protected from danger and can avoid physical pain. They are surrounded by armed guards, and they travel in bullet-proofed cars. When their countrymen go to war the leaders stay at home and think, no longer riding into battle at the head of the army as Henry V did. Like the gods of old, the heroes have faded away and we are left wondering who and what in the world can we look up to and admire. Bravery, advancing into the face of danger and pain, is no longer the prince of virtues. Cunning has taken its place. The winner is he who is the swiftest and the most devious in evading danger, not the one who faces it and survives.

In the days of chivalry children were educated to take risks and to withstand pain. When schools were opened, competitive sports were evolved in which children fought mock battles where one team, like an army, fought another. They were not supposed deliberately, sadistically, to inflict pain but they were trained to accept it, if it occurred, without complaint. The boys held up as heroes were the brave ones, but bravery was not the prerogative of the winners; the losers, by being brave, won as well.

All Britons in the age of Elegance admired "bottom". "God won't love those", they were told, "who won't strike out for themselves." Boxing was the national nursery of manliness, in which a gentleman was expected to be "a proper man with his fists" and know how to "clear a lane of men" with his "morleys". Thomas Asheton Smith, when Master of the Quorn, after a set-to in a Leicester street with a six-foot coal-heaver, clamped a raw steak on both his eyes and sent his prostrated opponent a five pound note, for being the best man who had ever stood up to him.

Britain's leaders came from the ranks of "gentlemen", a gentleman being expected to know the rules of the game. He must behave appropriately, with kindness, compassion and decorum, but he must also be valiant.

> All gentlemen knew that they must be brave, show no sign of panic or cowardice, be courteous to women and children, be loyal to their comrades and meet death without flinching.

How much of such behaviour was the gentleman's by nature is impossible to determine. Why do shepherds choose certain types of collie dogs to train to herd their sheep? The training is all-important, but the breed of dog is important too. My Old English Sheepdog was never taught to do so, but he herded our hens into their shed every night on his own.

From early childhood, children were taught both the rules and how to practise them. From the time a child could first sit on a horse he became involved in the field sports of the countryside.

As Sir Walter Scott wrote of his countrymen:

> It gave them a strong and muscular character, saving them from all sorts of causeless fears and flutterings of the heart. Men who rode to hounds, shot duck in wintry marshes with breech-loaders, fished for salmon in moorland streams, learned, as boys, to snare and kill wild-fowl, snakes, hares, rabbits, badgers and all sorts of game and vermin, and

continued to do so whenever they had a chance so long as they could walk or stride a horse, were not likely to fail for lack of courage.

Asheton Smith said of hunting, "Throw your heart over and your horse will follow".

Everyone has the potential to be courageous. Cowardice can either be trained out of a child or allowed to develop in him. The fearful person allows doubt and the anticipation of failure to govern him, he runs away from pain. The courageous person centres and conserves his energies, being free to direct them where and when they are needed, whether that may be against his enemies from without or against the enemy of self-doubt gnawing him from within.

Courage is a useful, practical, technical skill, invaluable in dealing with either physical or mental pain. If it is not inborn it can and should be developed. No suffering is worse than fear, and courage provides the antidote. The old training is that if you fall off a horse you get straight back up again, if you are involved in a car crash you drive again immediately. You never give fear time to build up and get a hold of you. At the Badminton horse trials thrown riders, even if they are injured, climb straight back on to their mount, ignoring the pain. On the polo field an injured rider is given a brief cheer as he rides back to join his team. It is taken for granted that this is what he will do.

And it is not just "stiff upper lip" nonsense, but very practical common sense. It the rider has time to give his imagination free reign and to anticipate all the horrors to which he might be prey, he will be taken over by fear. No one can live happily if they are afraid.

I have great sympathy for those patients suffering from "anxiety neurosis", which is a euphemistic way of describing people who are a prey to panic. They lose contact with reality, the solid ground under the feet, and flounder in a world of fantasy fears which they have never been taught how to control. Throughout history, bravery in the face of pain or at the threat of death has been valued highly, not only among warriors but among saints as well. Courage stems from faith, from the ability to dispel doubt about the rightness of one's purpose or effort, and that faith is nurtured by training. The life style both of men-at-arms and religious is geared towards this end.

When King Henry VIII passed the Act of Supremacy, making him spiritual as well as temporal head of the Church in England, the Carthusian monks met in London to discuss the situation and how they should in conscience react to it. Henry insisted on their complete acceptance of the Act, and they refused to obey him. Three priors were arrested, found guilty of treason and sent to the Tower. They were kept there for a few days to allow their fears to develop, then they were lashed on to hurdles and dragged over the cobbled streets to the Tyburn, which is now Marble Arch. They were hanged, cut down before they were dead, and disembowelled.

One of the reasons for such barbaric treatment, which Henry knew would alienate him from the Pope and from many of his peers abroad, was to make such an example of these monks that their brethren would quickly submit. He underestimated both their courage and their faith. Three more were arrested and chained to pillars. It is said that the King himself visited them in an attempt to persuade them to accept his authority but they would not. They were hung, drawn and quartered. At any time during their imprisonment these men could have released themselves by submitting to the King, but they did not. They found the strength and the courage to withstand agonizing pain until death released them from it.

The Knights of Malta are members of a religious order originally founded to care for the sick among pilgrims visiting the Holy Land at the time of the crusades. In 1113 the Order was dedicated to St John the Baptist, and a hospital was set up in Jerusalem. Gradually the need to protect pilgrims from the attacks of the infidel changed the nature of the Order, which of necessity became more militaristic. Members were recruited from only the noblest families in Europe, and took monastic vows of chastity and obedience. As with all successful warriors, they were highly disciplined, trained to obey orders without question or doubt, and to put the good of the Order before all else. The finest of them all was said to be the Grand Master Jean Parisot de la Valette, after whom Valetta harbour in Malta is named. In his youth he was badly wounded in battle and lost his ship. He was captured by the Turks and sold as a galley slave.

Living as a slave was hardly living at all. Six men in a row were chained to a four-foot bench covered with sacking. Two officers, one in the prow, the other amidships, were armed with whips with which they flogged the prisoners mercilessly. They rowed sometimes for twenty hours at a stretch without rest of any sort. The officers put pieces of wine-soaked bread in their mouths to feed them, but if they collapsed, they were flogged to death, and thrown overboard like dogs.

For a year de la Valette survived this existence, and lived to escape and rejoin his brethren. He was seventy, a great age in those days, at the time of the siege of Malta, when under his leadership for four terrible months the Knights withstood an onslaught from the numerically superior forces of Suleyman the Magnificent. They suffered great deprivations but they won. It was said that to survive a year in the galleys a man must be incredibly tough. To survive a life of warfare and still be fit to lead his men to such a victory at the age of seventy, he must have been almost superhuman.

De la Valette joined the Order as a child, and was trained to develop courage. His faith was such that neither pain nor physical hardship could defeat him. The only disaster would have been defeat itself.

St Ignatius Loyola (founder of the Society of Jesus, often better known as the Jesuits) was a soldier and trained his brethren by conditioning them to bravery, as he had been conditioned. At one time I was asked to teach a group of Ignatian-trained novices and their novice mistress about relaxed concentration and its application to prayer. I told them about the traditional importance given to posture in prayer, and how in the East yogis sit in the lotus posture while praying, so that the balance of the body eases the flow of breathing which can restrain the wandering mind.

In this position, sitting cross-legged on the floor, one foot is lifted on to the opposite thigh, and then the other, so that instead of the legs being crossed under each other they are crossed over the top. Anyone unused to it finds this way of sitting extremely painful to get into, to stay in, and particularly to get out of. When I was training I learned more about acute pain from sitting in the lotus position than from anything else.

The Jesuit-trained novice mistress was a wonderful, tough, middle-aged Irish woman determined that, if good could be wrought from anything, she would wring it. But when she sat down and crossed her legs her knees remained stubbornly up in the air, and try as she would, she could not flatten them sufficiently to get her feet over the top. She sat there in her black dress pressing down both knees with each hand, puffing and blowing in frustration. At last she called, "Sisters, will you come here" and as her two young novices approached she told them to stand, one on her right knee, one on her left, stamping them down to the ground. It took all my protestations to get her to realize that middle age is not the best time to start forcing one's legs into the lotus position.

The prospect of pain meant nothing to this lady. She did not control it by relaxing and riding with it as I did, she simply forbade it to impinge on her. She dared it to attack her. There was an element not only of furious determination but also of foolhardiness in her attitude.

In another case, Father Vincent McNabb, an English Dominican, in his old age removed his socks and shoes to gambol in the snow outside the church, saying afterwards that he did it to get his feet warm: "The colder you get, the warmer you feel."

Going forward bravely to meet adversity with no hesitation and with no doubt brings you safely through it. We used to know this but it has been forgotten. Now we must re-learn it.

7

Hospices and
Pain Relief Units

Two institutions make pain control their specialty, and both have been developed during the past thirty years. The Pain Relief Unit is a specialist unit attached to a general hospital, the best of them now are multi-disciplinary, employing anaesthetists, neurologists, psychologists, and physiotherapists who are detailed to teach relaxation therapy as well. Such units flourish in most health authorities, seeing patients referred by their GP or consultant whose pain, whatever it might be, is uncontrolled.

The second institution is the hospice. This movement started in England when Dame Cicily Saunders recognized the need of specialist care for patients in hospital who were beyond the help of invasive therapy. These patients are an embarrassing reminder of failure to the hospital doctor. His job is to cure, and when all hope is gone, his role is ambivalent. The burden of care then falls on the nurses, who have no authority to prescribe drugs, who are exceptionally busy, and who have neither the time nor the training to accompany their patients along the road towards death. The easiest course is to prescribe so much sedation that the patient is relieved of distress, but unfortunately even this procedure has problems. Drugs produce side-effects which are themselves distressing: constipation, liver or kidney failure, emphysema, all of which can be a direct cause of death. In 1978 Dame Cicily wrote:

We should aim for the relief that enables a patient not only to die peacefully but also to LIVE until he dies, as himself and not as what has been termed "an uncomplaining residue".

The ethos in a modern hospital is similar to that in the service bay of a modern garage. The patient is a mechanism which is malfunctioning in some respect. He has to wait his turn until eventually he is put on the hoist for inspection and, depending on the result, referred for treatment. The more medicine becomes a business, the more this attitude will prevail, despite the tradition of care in the health service.

In a garage, when a car is beyond repair it is towed to the scrapyard for re-cycling. In a hospital it is not so simple, and the incurable patient becomes an embarrassment to all concerned. If he is just crippled he can be released into the care of the social services. If he is in continual pain he does not disappear so easily. If he is dying, now, through the work of Dame Cicily, he can be sent to a hospice.

The most distinctive aspect of a hospice is the difference in the attitude of the staff. They are there to serve the patient in all his needs. If he wants to talk, a nurse or an auxiliary nurse will be detailed to stay with him. If he just wants someone to hold his hand he can call for this too. Pain relief is given priority.

Dame Cicily wrote in 1977:

Successful symptomatic treatment should enable a patient to be so relieved of physical distress that he is freed to concentrate on other matters. If we are to overcome the sense of failure which tends to pervade the atmosphere which surrounds the dying, we need to be aware of the proper criterion of success in this situation. It is not to be seen primarily in our activities but rather in what the patient and his family can achieve in the face of progressive physical deterioration. This may be the most important part of his life, and the spirit often becomes stronger and more individual as the body weakens.

In a general hospital, if the existence of the spirit is recognized at all, the patient is referred to the chaplain, whose training may be in reciting prayers rather than in relieving suffering.

A hospice is not only a place of care for the dying. Many patients with extensive disease still live for many years, and the hospice is devoted to enhancing the quality of this life, many of them having flourishing out-patient departments. Hospices differ in appearance from general hospitals. The floors are carpeted so that the sound is different. The entrance often has a box of cuddly toys for children to play with, and a comfortable room for patients and their visitors to sit in, with TV and refreshments.

One of the staff nurses or the sister welcomes the patient, and the admissions clerk is carefully chosen to take her place as a pleasant member of the staff, contrasting sharply with some of the boot-faced ladies sitting unmoving, hardly speaking, outside the ward of a general hospital, and who give the patient the first inkling of the new world he is entering and the low status of the role as a patient which he has to adopt.

The ratio of nurses to patients is sometimes one to one in a hospice, and the quality of the nurses volunteering for hospice work is usually very high. They are skilled at recognizing and assessing the patients' pain. They are also aware of contributory factors which exacerbate pain; if the patient is distressed because his children have not visited him, or if he is told that his prognosis is bad, his pain will intensify. In a general hospital staff time is at such a premium, and specialist opinion is so unco-ordinated, that these subtleties may go unrecorded.

In a hospice the staff are expert at dealing with the pharmacological aspects of pain, and can recognize the symptoms caused by pain-killing drugs – nausea, constipation, depression – and know that the level of toxicity needs to be brought down. When I worked in a hospice relaxation therapy was still an unknown quantity regarded with suspicion by some, but when the effects of the method were seen, it was often the nurses who observed their patients' tension and asked that they should be referred to me.

We were fortunate in that one of the nurses was a born comedian, a middle-aged woman with a bubbling wit. Even if the patient is dying there are still things to laugh about, and there is nothing more relaxing and pain reducing than laughter. There is no reason why, because a patient is dying, he should be treated as though he was already dead, being surrounded with a hush of gloom and despondency which isolates him even more from his fellow men.

One of the difficulties in staffing a hospice is in finding the balance between caring and sentimentality, laughter and brutality, sensitivity and preciousness. It is the old, old problem of the intrusive ego, and outsiders don't help. They say, "I don't know how you do it. You people working in this field are so wonderful. You are all angels. You are all saints." This is dangerous slush. The last thing dying patients need is to provide an ego trip for do-gooders.

The one quality needed in hospice staff is the ability to respect their fellow men and to be neither ambitious nor judgemental about them. All the usual moral difficulties present themselves. Does the end justify the means? If a patient is famous his treatment might provide the sort of publicity which will produce funds needed for more staff or more beds. Should he, therefore, receive more care and better attention than the others? The nurse looking after him might get her photo in the papers or on television. The death of the famous has great news value.

All sorts of moral judgements have to be avoided with the patients themselves. Nurses undertaking hospice work are often practising Christians, and it may be deeply offensive to find that their patient has no belief structure at all and that efforts to give him spiritual comfort are spurned.

Laughter is great value. Laughter among the staff at our fumbling attempts to help, at our or other people's self-importance, at the wonderful leveller that death is. Laughter among the patients at anything they can find to laugh about. Our patients liked to play bingo in the afternoon. Every sort of cultural option was offered to them – flower arranging, painting, lectures, film shows, but they wanted, and they got, bingo. They won prizes of Mars bars or bags of sweets, they laughed, they were in a noisy, normal atmosphere and that was what they wanted. It is some years since I was there and I wonder whether the bingo still exists? The hospice has expanded, and now has lecture rooms and staff rooms. The day unit is an architect's dream. It would certainly look better on reports to say that the patients are offered a variety of cultural activities rather than perpetual bingo. The social workers engaged there now replacing the nursing auxiliaries are educated ladies not comics. I wonder – and I'd love to know about the bingo.

Because the patients were happy and the atmosphere easy, our nurses had more opportunity to observe, to pick up any change in the patients' condition. If they withdrew from the others and looked worried or sad the nurses noticed and gave them the opportunity to confide. They were more than nurses, they were friends. If any patient seemed physically distressed a doctor was immediately on call.

The atmosphere in that unit was not of death but of laughter and life, and although patients died or deteriorated and were admitted to the ward, everything was done to prevent those who were left from becoming morbid or depressed about it. A chair which had been occupied for months or even years by a well-known friend would one day inevitably stand empty. But life and the process of dying goes on. The routine of the day, the laughter, the jokes, the bingo continued, muted perhaps but undaunted.

8

Mary and James

Pain has always fascinated me, maybe because my father was a doctor. I can't walk past someone in pain without feeling guilty if I don't stop to help. Sometimes, in the hospital, I walked on to the ward just at the right time, when one of my patients was having an intravenous injection or the lung aspirated. Very junior doctors are often allocated these jobs and they get nervous, particularly if it is the first time they have tried and if they are in front of an audience of tough nurses and a frightened patient. I start by relaxing the patient and the effect rubs off onto everyone else.

Anyone can relax when things are going well, but the time when relaxation is necessary and effective is when things get tough. It is then that we tighten up in self-protection, it is then that we cause ourselves damage, and make the pain and the whole procedure worse.

When I needed a job once I asked the medical director of a pain relief unit for the opportunity to work there with his patients, and he agreed. We talked at length about the need to work on the patients' reaction to pain; about how, for no apparent reason, two patients with the same clinical symptoms of injury will differ radically in their complaints about pain; about how there is no way of making an objective assessment – you can't stick a needle into the patient and say, "Yes. This patient has x degrees of pain." You have to judge by your own observation and by what the patient tells you.

It is very difficult. If there is no obvious cause for pain

the patient runs the risk of being diagnosed as hypo-
chondriachal. I have seen patients begging so persistently
for help that they have even undergone unnecessary
surgery. Yet when you do meet someone articulate and
able to co-operate fully with their treatment, it is a
pleasure.

One afternoon in the pain relief unit on the ward round
we came to the bed of a very vocal, middle-aged lady, a
lively, intelligent, strong personality with an obvious sense
of humour, although she was extremely nervous. She had
been admitted to have a nerve block to relieve her back
pain, but because of bad previous experiences she was
reluctant to go ahead without firm assurance that it would
help her condition, and also that it would do her no harm.
She was called Mary.

The doctors were non-committal with her, and we
discussed her case after the round. They were hesitant to
treat her because they could not, in all honesty, give her
the assurances she demanded. According to the rule-book
she should not have had her previous trouble – but she
had, and no one could guarantee that it would not happen
again. I suggested that I should see her and they were
delighted to agree; it let them off the hook – it might do
good, and in any case it could do no harm. Here is her
own report:

> The cause of my pain had been a growth on the roots
> of the nerves in the spinal cord. There had been ten
> years of steadily increasing pain until a mylogram
> x-ray finally clarified the diagnosis. During the final
> two years I had been unable to sit in a chair or to
> lie down for more than an hour at a time.
>
> Two lots of surgery in twelve months removed
> most of the growth, which was described as non-

111

malignant but persistent. Radio therapy treatment checked further growth but produced scar tissue which caused intense sciatic pain.

When I was admitted to the pain relief unit, apart from the physical pain I was prey to painfully emotive memories and fears arising from a disastrous epidural, after which I had been paralysed for many hours; a second mylogram – the first had been appallingly painful; a second spinal operation in exactly the same place as the first; no fear about cancer but deep fear about the effects of radiotherapy and the pain which resulted from it; three weeks' pain relief treatment in a hospice where the sight of a fellow patient in the opposite bed disturbed me greatly. She had been there for a year and was now paralysed and in great pain. The cause, I was given to understand, was the same spinal trouble as mine. I felt I was looking at my own future.

When I returned to the hospice as an out-patient some weeks later I was told that my fellow patient's case was not quite the same as mine, but was also told that my back trouble would almost certainly recur and that I would end up in a wheelchair. I was badly shaken by this news and tried, unsuccessfully, to find out how long I might have.

On my next out-patient visit the pains were much worse and I was referred to the pain relief unit for a possible nerve block. I had to wait three weeks for an appointment, during which time fears about the block built up. It seemed likely from all I could find out that it involved a spinal anaesthetic, and this triggered off the terror of a repeat of the epidural experience.

While I waited the congestion and spasms in

112

the tail of the spine increased. I had sciatic pains down my right leg, and what felt like semi-paralysis in both legs, which made walking very difficult. The wheelchair prediction seemed to be coming nearer.

As well as anxieties about my medical welfare I was worried on the domestic front, about whether I will be able to drive my car again. I live in an isolated, country village where a car is an essential. After the second operation I lost confidence completely and I am still trying to come to terms with the new driving technique, having had my car converted for a disabled driver.

I am worried about whether I will be able to handle my horse again after two years of parking him on friends. A horse has always been a deeply important therapeutic part of my life. I am able to accept the fact that my riding days are over, but, if I cannot drive him either, I will have to sell him. I will not keep an active working horse as a pet. This has been a cause of deep worry and distress.

I am worried about my profession as a writer. I have been working hard to rebuild my free-lance career. I really thought I was on the way last year as I was able to produce a book that involved a lot of desk work and travelling by car. If sitting at a desk becomes impossible I am intensely afraid that my future career will be in jeopardy.

The day after being introduced to the relaxing technique she wrote:

Although I am both interested and enthusiastic because it makes sense there are two initial obstacles to overcome:

1. An illogical feeling of embarrassment that it may not be possible for me to do what is expected.

2. The disentangling of previous associations with other relaxation techniques, i.e. Yoga and the seven centres learned from books, plus, long ago, a wartime memory of being taught relaxation on an ATS officer cadet course in a bitterly cold, unheated Brighton hotel. This consisted of lying flat on our backs on the freezing floor of what had been the ballroom and being told to make our foreheads "as smooth as a billiard ball", after which we went round each limb tightening the muscles and letting go. It had never occurred to me to wonder at the relevance of this to my job as an officer.

Now I am being asked, instead of tightening the muscles, to think or breathe down the inside of an arm. It is difficult to get mentally adjusted to withdrawing oneself from outside and to focus into a limb. The first lift-from-the-elbow movement is a self-conscious, done-from-the-outside affair. After two or three attempts, synchronized with breathing, the idea seems to take root. I find myself searching for my own set of words to describe what I am doing, but fail to do so.

Does the arm now feel different from the other?

Surprisingly enough, yes, it does.

What sort of different?

Difficult to describe. Perhaps "leaden" or "heavy" would be the word. I wonder if it's meant to feel like this.

We move down to the left leg.

This is surprising. I was expecting the right arm to be matched up first. I put up a mental block over this, and take some time to get adjusted to thinking down the left leg.

Drawing it up with the knee bent seems to be too much a conscious muscular movement. I feel I am reducing it to the forbidden level of a PT exercise. The relaxed leg is definitely more difficult to achieve than the forearm.

I'm told I am frowning. I wonder whether to break the deepening silence of relaxation by giving voice to the questions and comments that flit through the mind as it is stimulated by the teaching and tries to absorb this new knowledge.

As we move over to the right leg I realize that I've tensed up my shoulder muscles. Wonder why? Am I still resentful because the right arm has not been attended to in the "logical" order of "arms and legs"? The four limbs are dealt with, and an inert body lies very much aware of its weight pressing down on the bed.

One of the best moments is the utter stillness at the end of each out-breath when lungs and stomach are collapsed on to the spine – or so it feels. There is a blissful inertia until one has to make the effort to breathe in again. A tempting speculation arises about whether one could bring one's life to a peaceful end by simply ceasing to breathe.

The next session was with a fellow patient in a side room, and Mary found both the privacy of being away from the ward and the companionship created a much better atmosphere.

As it was his first and my third session I was happy to be on the sideline and to stop wondering whether to respond in speech. My fellow patient obviously had no such concerns, and we both remained totally silent, which was a great help to concentration, though I wondered what the absence of reaction did for our teacher.

Lying on a polished floor also made the leg movement much easier sliding it up and down.

I particularly liked the introductory analogy of the breathing rhythm to the surge and drop of a sea wave – an analogy specially geared for my deep-sea trawlerman companion. His immediate response could be sensed in the silence.

I find it particularly difficult to relax my face and features. I am very aware that in daily life I screw up my face at the least provocation, especially when involved in any sort of demanding physical effort. I wonder if I still twitch my nose when I am tense? It had become such an ingrained habit that I remained unaware of it unless I asked friends to tell me.

"When we are anxious we grit our teeth."

Damn it. I'm gritting mine right now. My jaw is all tensed up. I attend to this and wonder what other bits of me have escaped my attention. I find a tensed up muscle in the left thigh. Every time I think I'm relaxed I find more tension. This is going to be a long job.

It is plain from the way she approached the therapy that this lady was both intelligent and honest. If I were to say which qualities were the most important in assessing the ability to learn this therapy, I would say courage and honesty. Tension is a part of the protective mechanism of the body, letting it go means that you allow yourself to be vulnerable. You FEEL vulnerable. Lying flat on your back on the floor with your eyes closed you ARE vulnerable. Anyone could step on your face before you knew it. Even releasing tension and letting your arm fall requires courage. Many people find it very difficult to do even such a simple, safe movement as lifting the forearm and letting it fall back to the floor. Courage is not innate, but it is a quality which can and should be developed. It is the basis of every virtue.

As I grow older I find myself increasingly impatient with dishonesty – time is too short. Anyone unable or unwilling to face the truth about themselves has not even reached first base. I use a video camera to back up my judgement of a person's state of tension. From it they can see objectively where incorrect posture causes tension, where self-consciousness induces jerky, awkward movement, where pain is exaggerated by sympathetic, unnecessary tension in other parts of the body.

Mary had a successful epidural within two days, and is now, ten years later, mobile and happy, writing, driving her horse and using her car. I asked her how things were going and she wrote back:

> When I went home from the Pain Relief Unit I took the Fleming relaxation tape and a broomstick. The tape has been lent to many friends, the broomstick is still my daily companion.
>
> Every day about lunchtime I lie flat on the floor to let my spine go down. It is only by lying flat on my back that I realize to what extent tension, of which I am unaware, has caused the spine to arch like a croquet hoop, producing all kinds of night cramps and other discomforts. I can now even lie full length on the broomstick and go fast asleep!
>
> Twenty minutes' total relaxation in this way makes an incredible difference to the remainder of the twenty-four hours. I get from it peace of mind as well as peace of the body.

I taught Mary to lie on a broomstick for three reasons: to help her to understand her reaction to pain; to flatten out the tension in her spine; and to help her to concentrate.

She made suggestions for the future:

1. A trained team of relaxation therapists to spread the work.
2. A telephone organization on Samaritan lines for follow-up therapy from home.
3. A tape geared for people-in-pain issued through hospitals only, to protect it from the greedy hands of pirate predators ready to cash in on people's sufferings.

James

I was first told about James at a case conference we held each day at the hospital where I worked. He was the biggest problem of the moment.

He had cancer of the bowel, and various procedures had only temporarily arrested the progress of the disease. Nothing more could be done for him, and the purpose of his admission was to stabilize a regime of pain control. He was forty-five and had gone from a poor start in life to be a successful executive. He was unhappily married and had three children.

They said that he complained of pain in his feet, abdomen and side, he sobbed continually and he would accept no comfort. He had to be moved from the main ward to a private room because he upset other patients. He would stand at the foot of the bed of a quietly-dying patient, staring at him with great mournful eyes, like the ancient mariner at the wedding feast.

They told me that it was not easy to form any relationship with him. Like many others in his position, he resented and was angered by the health of those around him. The staff thought it very doubtful whether he would accept my intervention, but he was already on a high dose of analgesics and on heavy tranquillizers so there was nothing else they had to offer. Both he and his wife had already seen a psychiatrist, which had only aggravated the situation, and both swore they would never repeat the experience.

I went to his room in some trepidation. I remember pausing outside and thinking, "My God! Why do I set myself up like this? I don't HAVE to do it."

He was blank-faced when I went in, looking at me with no change of expression. I didn't waste time on preliminaries, but asked him to lie down on the bed, to close his eyes and to bring his attention back to his body in its present situaition; to let go the tension which pervaded his whole being. After ten minutes I could see an improvement as I talked. I stopped, and he opened his eyes, acknowledging that he felt easier. This deeply impressed, almost shocked, him. I had not touched him. No invasive treatment had been used; yet he was better.

He recognized that there was a chance that he could contribute towards relieving his own condition, and when I saw him on the next and the following day I was delighted to find that he approached his training as he would a job of work, and worked hard at it. He reported back his discovery of previously unrecognized tensions and occasions when, although he still became up-tight, he was able to calm down and control himself.

On the fourth day he was discharged, pain-controlled. But he was afraid to go home – he didn't know how he would cope without his job, and he had alienated his friends by telling them too bluntly that he was dying. Understandably, such a statement is an embarrassment and a conversation-stopper when playing Scrabble or bridge at a supposedly casual social evening. The friends didn't come back.

Seeing his children made him cry.

I suggested that as well as following the regime of drugs he must structure his days at home. He must use the discipline of relaxation, listening to the tape I gave him at least twice a day. He must remember it also in his activities during the day, so that whenever he felt overwhelmed by fear or by grief or by pain, he should stop still and see what he could do about relieving his own agony. Instead of giving way to it he should relax, come back into the reality of his present situation, come "Back to his senses", realizing that grief is for loss of the future and regret for the past, and that all these churning emotions only served to exacerbate his pain. He should occupy himself with anything that he found interesting. He must fill his mind and divert his thoughts with any occupation that he found pleasant.

He practised constantly. Never, from the word go, did I have to motivate James to work. As soon as he saw results from what I was suggesting he gave it all the enthusiasm and energy that he could. From the first day, he wanted to report on his discoveries – how he had tried out this or that procedure to see what he could accomplish by himself.

Such a student is a delight for any teacher, and I must admit that in my experience men are better at working than women. Once they get past the initial embarrassment they work for the results they want, whereas women are sometimes too passive, expecting the results to happen, to come as a gift.

After his discharge I heard no more from James until about six weeks later, when he was re-admitted. The disease had spread and he was in acute pain. He had a blockage in the bowel for which he might, or might not, require a colostomy operation.

He was a different person, friendly, quite calm and helpful to the other patients. His bed was back in the main ward and the man next to him was dying. James led him around, took him for walks, laughed and joked with him and they became great friends.

He told me that he had done exactly as we had planned. He had brought back with him an armful of crossword and other word-game puzzles. Though it would have been a penance for me to do them, his mathematical mind enjoyed it and they "passed the time". He listened to the tape conscientiously each day, and I never needed to give him encouragement to practise. He always practised.

Although he was in pain he was not distressed, but a few days later the pain escalated and he was rushed to theatre, where an emergency colostomy was performed. I saw him next day and he was very proud: he had been able to support his wife through the traumas of the previous evening, and had been calm and confident where she had been near hysteria.

The colostomy worked well and things settled down peacefully until, inexplicably, the pain recurred. This happened on a Saturday and I was telephoned to come and see him. Again he had a blockage and this time James was in total panic. His eyes stared out of a twitching face and his body was rigid with terror. He could do nothing to help himself, and we had to start right back at the beginning again. He had to prove to himself, from his own experience, that he was making himself worse by the way he was reacting to the new situation. I stayed with him for three hours and, at last, he relaxed, calmed down, and the pain immediately eased. His bowel then started to function again.

That evening was a time of great rejoicing for him and his family. The experience he had been through gave him confidence that he could relieve his own stress even in the worst conditions. He accepted that the disease was progressive and that nothing could halt its progress, but that the problems it caused and the pain he suffered were exacerbated by his own hypertension. When he relaxed his body functioned and adapted as well as it possibly could.

I gave him a personalized cassette player to use, because although he was more than willing to practise relaxation he could not be expected to practise it non-stop. I chose tapes of music to give him with great care, and changed them as time went on. The earphones relay the sound directly into the head so concentration becomes easy. The music blocks out discursive thoughts or disturbing emotions.

It had to be gentle music for my purpose – no loud, angry pop. It could be lively but it must not be distressing. Although he was no musician he liked Mozart when he heard it for the first time, and to lighten him and make him laugh, I gave him music from the Greek islands, dancing music, utterly from the gut, charming and funny.

He enjoyed it very much and listened more and more to the tapes. He was confined to bed now, but he practised relaxation every morning and the staff and the patients knew that they must leave him alone during this time, letting him find and enjoy his own tranquillity. He said to me one day, "It's peace. It's all peace."

He set himself short term goals: he wanted to live until Christmas (it was now late November), and he wanted to see his children again. His wife had forbidden them to visit their father for fear it might upset them. She came every night, although her home was a long distance away and she had to rely on friends to drive her, but she would not allow her children to come and they had not been told that their father was dying. We had to work on her as well, to make her realize that she could not deny the children the right to see their father, or him the right to see them. The results, after his death, could well destroy her relationship with her children.

As James became gentler and more understanding things got better, and it was decided that they should all spend Christmas together. I was away but I heard what a marvellous time they had. The sick neighbour and his family were there and they all celebrated together.

After that James wanted to live until his birthday, six weeks later. A week beforehand he had a pulmonary embolism and found he could not breathe. Whereas when things were going well, I could leave him to work on his own, in times of emergency he needed my support.

One day on going into the ward I heard a strange noise, and when I looked at his bed saw it shaking as he writhed on top of it. He was white, without colour of any sort, his teeth were chattering and every part of his body was rigid. He was in a rigor. Once again I stayed with him, calming him, telling him to breathe out, to feel the weight of his body going down to the bed, to come back to the core of stability inside himself. The nurse had gone to fetch him hot water bottles and blankets, but when she returned they were not necessary, he was calm and relaxed again.

He deteriorated gradually, peacefully after this. He knew he was near to death but he could put the thought of it away from him by coming back into awareness of reality, awareness of the present. He had the key to entering another dimension of time. We live in the past or the future, looking back over the things that have happened in the past or waiting for the things to come. He learned to live in the present, to value every moment of time, and by focusing on that, to be unafraid.

He died, gently, three weeks later.

He practised no religion. I admired him for his honesty when he said, "I haven't practised religion during my life. I'm not going to call a priest now because I am afraid", but he knew that the sense of peace he felt was in some way a reflection of God.

In the Christmas week that I was away I left him with tapes to carry him through, and the following is the transcript of one. He had already learned how to relax and to concentrate. He knew how to reach into another dimension. It even had a special colour for him – mauve with gold edgings, like a storm cloud covering the sun. I was in the tape reminding him of things he knew already.

JAMES'S TAPE

First of all, close your eyes. This isn't just to cut off from outside, but to give yourself room to listen to your other senses so that the sense of vision does not take priority over them.

Each one of us has an inside person and an outside one. What goes on inside is completely alone, and when you close your eyes you are relating to this "I" which is alone in all of us. It is alone and yet, because it is identical in every one of us, it is never alone.

When you open your eyes after being in this area inside yourself, you have to change. You have to put on a mask for other people. It is really for their good. Each person you know wants you to play a different role for them; you play the husband for your wife; you play the father for your children; you play the entertainer for your friends; to each you give a different aspect of yourself.

But, because the inside self does not change, it needs no protective mask. So, when your eyes are closed, look into darkness. Don't try to imagine what may be going on around. And you do this by relaxing your eyelids, your eyebrows and the muscles around your eyes.

Feel the difference in the texture – how soft your eyeballs are and how gentle compared with the hardness of the bone.

Feel the air come in through your nose and mouth. Feel how it vibrates through your lips. And follow the path of the air as it comes into your face and then on into your head. Let it go right up to the top of your head as though it were cleaning it out of all tension. And then it goes down through the back of your head, feeling the touch of the pillow, through the back of your neck, past your back until it finds its home in your diaphragm. This is where it grows from and where it comes back to in an ebb and flow of movement.

When breathing is shallow, when it is disturbed, it is like the little, angular waves on the surface of a choppy sea. When you let go and breathe out it becomes like the deep sea swell miles under the surface, where the water lifts you up and down as you go with it. Even if it feels as though you are being sucked into a whirlpool, go with it. Don't resist. You will find calm again.

Follow your breathing then, until it extends into your arms and legs. Lift your arms and let them fall. Lift them with the swell of your breathing. Notice how, as you breathe in, your arm becomes lighter. Feel, really become engulfed in, this feeling of lightness. Feel the pull away from gravity, away from the earth. And then the inside-outness as you breathe out again and become heavy.

Notice too how, when you breathe in like this, you don't

become so hot. The heat drains away. And always accept what you feel without fear. "O.K. This is what it is like to feel hot. So what?"

It doesn't MATTER whether you feel hot or not. You can leave all that to the doctors and the nurses. It is their job to work out the reasons and to gauge the significance of it. It could even be because they keep the ward extremely hot. Or it may be that your heat-regulating mechanism has gone a bit haywire. There is nothing you can do about it now except to accept it and relax. Then it will be better.

Let your breathing go down through your body, and don't by-pass any part of it. Don't think of your body as though it belonged to the other, the external "I", the "I" which is apparent to other people, the "I" which is always in competition, wondering whether it functions as well as other bodies do.

Feel it from inside and don't resent it because it has let you down. We all have to forgive our bodies. All of us would like to be superman or superwoman – beautiful and strong and healthy. We have to forgive our body that it is not so exalted, particularly when it has caused pain. Then we treat it like an enemy, a traitor.

You can track this feeling by recognizing how breathing avoids the pain. Try not to do this but to breathe right through your pain. Feel compassion for your body for having got itself into such a state.

Every part of you must take part in breathing – every part. It is only when we are blinded by the rules of convention that we identify this part as good and that part as hidden and secret and rather horrible. Let breathing glow freely through your whole body.

Breathe into your legs now. Feel how there is nothing expected of them. They don't have to lie in wait for activity. Let them rest. Feel their weight and their warmth. Don't imagine what they look like from outside. You must have given them a hard time for quite a while for them to be as tense as this. Let them rest. And your feet. And your toes. And the sole of your foot too. Notice whether you can feel your feet tingle, as sometimes you can feel your hands tingle. Feel the warmth going into them from your breathing. Feel the ebb and flow, the swell of breathing lifting your whole body, even to your feet.

Then, go back to the centre. Notice whether you feel not only the colour but the shape of your breathing pattern too. To me it is always like a figure of eight. It goes across my body and up one side and into my head. Then it swings down across to the other side and through the centre like the gate in a car's gear box. When it reaches the diaphragm it is in neutral, but "neutral" does not mean "nothing". It is an enormously positive place. It cannot be described as this or that. It is just itself.

Then your breath goes down through into your legs and feet; and then comes back to the centre again.

Your breathing shape may well be different from mine. Everybody is different and unique. The thing to avoid is the jagged up-down, up-down rhythm, like soldiers marching on parade. Relaxed breathing describes a curve, both at the top and at the bottom.

Notice too whether the colour of breathing changes, whether it gets brighter or paler as it flows through your body.

Listen to it all the time and watch it. In one breath you can encompass all experience. Nichola of Cusa said that movement is "rest drawn out in an orderly series" and "the maximum is equal to the minimum".

One breath is all breath. It is time present. Time present contains all time. Feel each moment of time like a drop of rain as it comes to you. It is not what you do with time

127

that matters; it is the very essence of time itself.

We are so concerned with what we do – running round like demented hens competing with each other. Being is all that matters – no more. Let go into being, into the true reality of one's own being. And it never ends. There is no time that any one of us can say, "I know it all". Each breath is a progression into greater and deeper understanding. And peace.

PART THREE

9

Blaming God

Once I believed that thinkers were men or women who sat in ivory towers in Oxford or Cambridge, arguing endlessly about less and less important things. The truth is quite different: they have much power. They may live among towers but these people dictate the way our society is run and the attitudes we have towards it.

I lived in Oxford or thereabouts for many years, and I heard discussions where conflicting opinions were presented about new ideas originating from anywhere in the world. A very long time afterwards I heard these same ideas, from one side or the other, presented as gospel truth by sociologists, psychologists, Hampstead intellectuals or teachers, and then, later still, they permeated down the line and I recognized the same influences in women's magazines or in newspaper articles.

Thinkers are important because eventually their ideas, which we take over, often subconsciously and below the level of rational appraisal, affect the way we, as individuals, assess the practical problems of our lives. Pain is one of these problems.

Professional thinkers, those who are paid to think, claim authority by virtue of the objectivity of their thought reaching out towards the truth, and to justify their payment, but the multiplicity of opinions presented as objective truth by these professionals demonstrates that this is an impossible ideal. When faced with the problem of pain affecting us personally we would do well to start thinking it out for ourselves.

Myself when young did eagerly frequent
Doctor and Saint and heard great argument
About it and about: but evermore
Came out by the same door where in I went.

We are imprisoned by the conditioning which fetters our minds, and our opinions are not of our own making. They are ideas filtered down originally from the thinkers, but diluted and adulterated on the way until they reach us in whatever form we find palatable, either from a newspaper or from discussion with our peers, from reading a book or from watching television. If the person talking to us looks pleasant and possesses that strange quality "charm", we are more likely to adopt his views than if he is ugly and talks with a lisp.

So much for objectivity!

Pain is a subject which is rarely discussed, let alone discussed objectively. Our prejudices about pain have been allowed to take root and grow as uncontrolled as weeds. The subject is too vast, too unwieldy and yet too personal. It is a dangerous subject for anyone to tackle because a change in attitude can so easily be put to the test. Most opinions, no matter how extreme or conflicting, are allowed to flourish if their supporters so wish because there is no objective truth against which they can be measured. The objective truth about attitudes to pain relief is only too easy to put to the test: the pain either goes away or it stays.

The way we react to the impact of pain, whether of the mind or the body, depends on what our concept of pain is and how this concept fits into our world view. We cannot afford, when confronted by the reality of suffering, to have our thinking about pain smothered by prejudices which have grown up as weeds around half-digested ideas.

In 1962 a psychologist, Buytendijk, said that pain "is

not merely a problem but a mystery . . . A senseless element of life. It is a *malum* placed in opposition to life, an obstacle and a threat, which throws man aside like some wretched creature who dies a thousand times over again.''

This is the view about pain which, if we think about it at all, is the one most widely held. Its implications are far-reaching, extending into the realms not only of psychology but of philosophy and religion as well.

The difference between a problem and a mystery is that a problem is capable of solution, whereas a mystery is beyond solving. If Buytendijk is right – and he is only voicing what the majority think – so far as tackling pain is concerned we are defeated before we even start. If we are to agree that pain is wholly negative, wholly evil, if it is really ''senseless'', meaning unredeemable chaos, attacking without rhyme or reason, then the whole structure of religious belief is threatened, not only in the West but in the East as well.

If pain is a *malum* then Christians are in trouble, for how can a ''good'' God inflict senseless suffering on His creatures? This is the question always raised in the hospital where I work when I say I am a practising Catholic.

One answer proposed centuries ago is that God is not good. There are two co-eternal principles: one the good, the creator of spirit; the other, the bad, the creator of matter. This dualism was the central tenet of many heretical sects, and the trinitarian doctrines of Christianity, wherein opposites can be reconciled and paradox acknowledged, were rejected by them.

The heresy recurs again and again throughout history. Where can this mysterious *malum* arise if not from some evil principle? If this is so then, just as the freedom to choose between good and evil is denied, so our personal ability to transform pain is brought into question. We have no freedom, we have no choice.

There is no alternative, but, like a drowning man, to grab at any help that we can find from outside ourselves, from drugs, from any thing or person who will act as an analgesic agent – even though we kill ourselves in the process.

Marco Pallis, my teacher, presented an explanation in the chapter "Is there a problem of evil?" of his book *The Buddhist Spectrum*, where he describes the story of Adam and Eve, "than which no more illuminating symbolic narrative is to be found in all sacred literature".

Apologists who have wished to defend God against the accusation of being "the author of evil" – and many have been constrained so to defend Him – have missed one vital point: the paradise (of Adam and Eve) happy as it was, CONTAINED THE SERPENT . . . If one pauses to look closely into the premises of creation, one must surely wake up to the truth that a paradise, any paradise, MUST CONTAIN THE SERPENT . . . the perfection of a paradise without the presence of the serpent would be the perfection not of paradise but of God Himself. It would be, in sufic terms, "the paradise of the Essence". Therefore when one says of a paradise or anything else that is created good or perfect, this can only mean that it is good or perfect AS FAR AS PARADISE or any other created thing is able to be perfect.'

Moreover the same principle will apply in the case of a hell. A hell, to be a hell, must contain a trace of the TREE OF LIFE concealed in it somewhere; it cannot be a place of absolute evil or absolute imperfection or absolute anything. That is why, in the Tibetan iconography, for instance, when hells are depicted, a Buddha is always shown there, as a necessary, if latent, witness to the omnipresent truth.

Pain cannot be unmitigated evil. From the ideal state, before the intervention of suffering, there existed the possibility of pain, and this may have been at the time of Adam and Eve or it may occur when each child leaves the womb. Thinking of pain as totally evil can only make us despair and panic (which makes our suffering worse), or fight to avoid pain at all costs (which leads to an unhappy, materialistic society such as ours is now).

These are the attitudes which anyone working in pain relief has to fight, because thinking in this way makes the pain of the sufferer infinitely worse, and he is defeated before he starts. They are the attitudes implicit in the reaction of most patients, and they are based on superstition. Rudyard Kipling described them in his poem "Natural Theology":

PRIMITIVE
I ate my fill of a whale that died
And stranded after a month at sea . . .
There is a pain in my inside.
Why have my Gods afflicted me?
Wow! I am purged till I am a wraith!
Ow! I am sick till I cannot see.
What is the sense of Religion and Faith?
Look how the Gods have afflicted me.

PAGAN
How can the skin of a rat or mouse hold
Anything more than a harmless flea?
The burning plague has taken my household
Why have my Gods afflicted me?

All my kith and kin are deceased,
Though they were good as good can be.
I will out and batter my family priest,
Because my Gods have afflicted me.

MEDIAEVAL

My privy and well drain into each other
After the custom of Christendie . . .
Fevers and fluxes are wasting my mother,
Why has the Lord afflicted me?
The Saints are helpless for all I offer –
So are the clergy I used to fee.
Henceforward I keep my cash in my coffer,
Because the Lord has afflicted me.

MATERIAL

I run eight hundred hens to the acre.
They die by dozens mysteriously . . .
I am more than doubtful concerning my Maker.
Why has the Lord afflicted me?
What a return for all my endeavour –
Not to mention the L.S.D.!
I am an atheist now and for ever,
Because this God has afflicted me!

PROGRESSIVE

Money spent on an Army or Fleet
Is homicidal lunacy . . .
My son has been killed in the Mons retreat.
Why is the Lord afflicting me?
Why are murder, pillage and arson
And rape allowed by the Deity?
I will write to *The Times*, deriding our parson
Because my God has afflicted me.

CHORUS

We had a kettle, we let it leak;
Our not repairing it made it worse.
We haven't had any tea for a week . . .
The bottom is out of the Universe.

CONCLUSION

This was none of the good Lord's pleasure
For the spirit He breathed in Man is free,
But what comes after is measure for measure,
And not a God that afflicteth thee.

Pain has a positive role to play in our lives and in our ability to learn and develop.

We try to externalize misfortune, and the law of cause and effect, so familiar in Buddhism, is often bypassed in the West. There are rules governing our chance of survival. On an individual level, if we eat too much of sweet foods we vomit; on a world level if we poison plants and then eat them we die. There is no point in blaming God or any externalized *malum*. We are responsible for our own reactions, to pain as to any other thing.

The Christian belief is that there is but one God and He is good. It is we who must change, not God, we must transform evil into good, pain into peace. We will never be wholly successful – we will never be wholly anything – but we can at least try.

When faced with death, time and time again patients say, whether they are atheists or not, "Why has God done this to me?" They see their pain and suffering as a punishment and God as an avenger – the view of Buytendijk. If pain is a punishment then we can only expect to endure it. We cannot overcome it.

This persistent heresy is certainly one reason why we

don't think about pain calmly and sensibly. We feel an underlying sense of guilt when we have pain – "I must have done something dreadful to deserve such a punishment". We are also angry – "Why has this happened to me? Why didn't it happen to the man across the road? The one who looks and acts so appallingly?" We feel helpless – "I can usually control my life. What is happening now? I am like a child. I can't even get out of bed." We feel, more than anything, afraid. The world, which we have reduced in size and contained in a framework we can understand and manipulate, has suddenly burst its bounds and become uncontrollable chaos.

So we turn to the professionals, to doctors, nurses, psychologists, to provide a new and safer background; we think that they KNOW what causes our pain, they understand it all, they can be left to deal with it. If we lose control, if we start screaming or writhing around in agony on the floor, as many do, we will be given sedation, we won't embarrass anybody. Surely this is so?

It is not so. Uncontrolled pain is chaos, and medical staff are as afraid when they see it as anyone else.

Philosophy, the search for wisdom, for an understanding of the dilemmas we face, is not the concern only of the faceless brains of Oxford or Cambridge. Pain is a great leveller, and when it strikes they are as helpless as anyone else, they too are forced to come back into their bodies. When Wittgenstein was dying he asked for a Catholic priest to talk to him, specifying that he should be a man of faith rather than a professional philosopher. The anthropologist Levi-Strauss says that "Scientists do tolerate uncertainty and frustration because they must. The one thing they do not and must not tolerate is disorder . . .'

Uncontrolled pain on a ward, freely expressed, is

intolerable to everyone. John was a young man of thirty, struck down by a fatal disease in the prime of life. He had been unexpectedly successful in his career as an engineer, and for the past few years he had enjoyed the fruits of success, travelling, coming back to a wife and two children, living in a luxury home.

A young, attractive man dying makes a more exciting impact than the worn out old wrinklies with which hospitals usually abound, and the staff react accordingly. They home in on the young one, and no matter how the wiser staff members try to guide them, the younger ones empathize with their own generation. This doesn't always help the patient. Too many cooks spoil the broth and this is what happened to John. When I found that I couldn't get near him without interruption I backed off, and once I had taught him some of the relaxation technique, I kept away from him, until one day a doctor phoned to say that John was dying, but dying from uncontrolled fear. His physical condition was unchanged, and death should still be many months away but he had tachycardia: he could not breathe, he was panic-stricken. Unless help could be found, he would die before evening, as he was already on the highest possible level of sedation.

Long before I reached the ward I could hear him screaming. The atmosphere, instead of the usual calm cheerfulness, was grim. Everyone suffered with him, but the unending screaming was hair-raising. He was on his own now in a side room.

What had happened was that his condition had improved, and the psychiatrist, one of the many "cooks" called in to help him adjust to his situation, had suggested that he should be discharged into the care of his adoring mother, his wife and children, living two miles away, being "not suitable". On the first day John was fine. His mother wheeled him around in a wheelchair, fed him carefully and catered for his every need, as she had done when he was a baby. On the second day he collapsed. We never discovered whether there was any direct precipitant, but by the time he was readmitted he was at death's door. He said he was in pain, but his greatest problem was that he was, literally, frightened to death of death.

Death is the ultimate fear. The fear of chaos, total loss of order or meaning. That is what death means to many people. Again I quote Levi-Strauss: "A native thinker says, 'All sacred things must have their place'. It can be said that being in their place is what makes them sacred."

To anyone believing in the sacred, believing that there is a harmony, a pattern to which we can conform, death has its appropriate place. It is not defeat. When the time for it arrives death must be accepted in the same way as pain.

It is useless and arrogant trying to impose your own beliefs on a dying person, but it is possible to be of practical help. You can show the patient how to control his panic. If then he finds his own source of harmony that is a bonus both for him and for you. John could only reach that state if I stayed with him, and I could not sit with him every hour of every day. He recovered sufficiently to walk out in the sun, but his panic returned and he died.

I have worked in a mental hospital, in Wimpole Street, in a rehabilitation centre, in monasteries and convents, in pain relief units, in schools, in hospices, in general hospitals. The medicals denigrate the influence of the spirit. The religious denigrate the influence of the body. Medicals over-use drugs and invasive therapies; religious exaggerate the powers of the spirit, at times confusing this with an over-emphasis on their own power. Witch-doctors have their uses but they achieve better results when they keep their own egotism out of it.

Now I want to set up a therapeutic centre at Lourdes where body, mind and spirit are equally cared for. There will be no talk of alternative therapies. We will be concerned with pain control and with improving the situation of the patient, increasing his mobility, helping to change his attitude, and giving him unconditional support for any length of time up to a month. Our group will include doctors and nurses, helpers and therapists.

Lourdes is a place of pilgrimage to Our Lady. There are not the same problems with the concept of Our Lady as there are with the concept of God – no one sees her as being judgemental. The colour chosen to represent her is blue, the colour of healing. She is filled only with compassion. Therefore people in pain trust, they are less afraid, and because they believe in her compassion they look forward with hope, not for a cure but for help. The self-limiting boundaries which go with stereotyped illness are removed.

At Lourdes we examine the third alternative, which is to grasp the nettle, dispel the myths, to see that pain is not an attack from some external, malignant force. It is a response we make which is, to some unquantified degree, within our control, to the distinctions between opposites. If we are aware of the reality of the Trinity and of the third alternative, we can handle pain.

10

Suspending Disbelief

Soon it will be fashionable to believe in God again, as happens now and again. Politicians realize that the concept of God the Avenger lends pungency to the acceptance of the moral code, and scientists and philosphers murmur now about newly discovered proofs.

I need no further proof than the knowledge that there is a harmony which reconciles opposites, in which there is no distinction between opposites, and that this knowledge is available to us all. The living proof is that there can be peace in pain.

Lourdes used to be a small village in the Pyrenees, but it is now a bustling town selling expensive merchandise. Over a hundred years ago an adolescent, asthmatic girl, daughter of a poverty-stricken ex-miller, went to gather wood across the Gave river, but could not keep up with her sister and friend because her breathing was so bad, and, as she waited, she saw a lady standing in the cave above her.

She saw the apparition eighteen times and was instructed to scrape the ground for water. She found a spring which was discovered to have healing qualities, and Lourdes has been a centre of pilgrimage for the sick ever since. They bathe in the water from the spring, they pray for healing at the blessing of the sick and at the torchlight procession which weaves in a criss-cross pattern over the square before the great Basilica each night.

They pray to The Lady, the Mother of God, who appeared to the girl, St Bernadette.

We don't expect to see visions. We don't expect miraculous cures, although some have been reported and accepted as such after meticulous research by the medical team.

We go, not because we don't know all the arguments against belief, we know all about the possibility of superstition or self-deception obscuring our vision, but there is at Lourdes, a living sense of harmony – not just people rubbing along well together, but real, true harmony. Immense crowds throng the domain, all moving gently, all in control, silenced by a whisper from the celebrant priest.

We have been trained, in the society in which we live, to disbelieve. Like Doubting Thomas, we deny anything which we cannot see or hear or feel.

At Lourdes, however, we have to decide. We have to commit ourselves either to belief or to disbelief. I have experienced disbelief, and I see it all about me in England, in the unhappy faces and unco-ordinated bodies moving around the streets. Comparatively, disbelief is, at first, an easy option. Belief is more difficult, requiring the use of different compartments of the brain, exercising the supra--rational rather than the rational or the sub-rational.

Relaxation can, if you wish, free the brain from the constrictions of rationality and its absorption with time future or time past. The focus of attention is then centred on reality, as shown through the re-awakened senses, the windows on to the world.

At Lourdes we must face the possibility that we are insane or grossly stupid. We sing into the empty air, we strip and sink into cold, spring water in concrete cubicles. Great, lovely buildings have been built to remind us of the apparition of a lady, THE lady, the Mother of God, the female cosmic principle, whatever way you wish to describe and interpret her – to an asthmatic peasant girl. We must face the possibility of insanity or crass stupidity but we must also face the possibility that it is all true.

The unbeliever has no knowledge other than the negatives. He has no conception of an awareness which is beyond the ordinary state of consciousness, because he accepts only those things which can be proved by a process of analysis. His God, his objective truth can be reached only by using the computer mechanism of his brain, the cortex, and so any knowledge reached through art or religion is inexplicably invalid.

Bernadette actually saw the lady, but Bernadette was a saint and a mystic. Scientists might declare her mad. I heard an eminent psychiatrist solemnly state that, were Jesus Christ to be born again he would be certified as schizophrenic and locked up for his own safety and for the safety of the community at large.

"The mystical view of consciousness is based on the experience of reality in non-ordinary modes of awareness", says Capra, a new scientist. Non-ordinary they may be, but they are available and within the reach of the most ordinary. If this were not so religious perception would disappear.

Bernadette was, for a time, a shepherdess, and lived in the country outside Lourdes, spending her days alone in the hills overlooked by the Pyrenees. The countryside there is strange and mysterious. Most of us are sensitive to holy places, and throughout history special places have been known as wonder-full. Delphi is one, and others the places where the Druids chose to build their circles of stone; so are certain churches and cathedrals; and Lourdes.

In our time we have become so mechanistic, so concerned with aggrandisement and barter that we lose the element of wonder – maybe because it is freely available to all. Wonder cannot be bought. We look at things and places, seeing only their "value" and whether, by exploiting them, we can accumulate more or exchange them for other things. I asked one of the local waitresses in a café in Lourdes whether she believed in The Lady. She smiled sadly and said, "No".

Lourdes, like Jerusalem, has plenty of time for both wondering and bartering, but nothing is allowed for sale on the Domain where the Grotto of The Lady is, and the Basilica. As we approach the Domain wonder comes into its own, and disbelief is suspended.

Bernadette's family were impoverished. The contrast between the beauty of the natural world in which she worked as a shepherdess and the squalor of her parents' room, a former prison cell in Lourdes, to which she returned, where the smoke from the open fire and the confined space in which the whole family lived aggravated her asthma, made no sense to her then as it makes no sense to us now. Why do some of us live in beauty and peace, whereas others live in filth and pain?

In different degrees we all face the same dilemma. The conditions in which we live may be less grim but pain, like the sting of a scorpion, does not discriminate between people; between the worthy and the unworthy; between the rich and the poor. Disease or loneliness cannot be assuaged by wealth alone.

Both the scientist and the psychic, the one using reason, the other prey to superstition, try to use their powers to ensure that the future moves in a predictable way.

With reason we barter with our lives, using the computer mechanism of the brain. It becomes like a huge betting shop where we calculate what the future may bring by working out the odds – "If I go out in the rain I may catch cold. Is it worth it?" "If I am subservient to the boss

145

he won't give me the sack. Is it worth it?'' "If I work from nine to five in a job I detest I can provide for my old age – if I live that long. Is it worth it?'' Reason calculates the odds and, on the basis of quantity, we are frequently right. But we can never be certain. There is no Absolute unless we accept that there is a God. The sun has risen so far every day of my life but that does not mean that one day the land will not remain dark.

The other negative is superstition, which tries to influence the pattern of the future but gets the connections wrong. The superstitious person may believe that by avoiding the cracks in the pavement he will attract good luck. You see superstition at work when tennis players bounce the ball x number of times before serving, and will wear only a lucky colour. If you are a bad player, wearing a different coloured shirt is not going to make you a good one. If you can't serve well, bouncing a ball fifty times first is not going to help you to get it over the net.

The truth is, we can never predict anything with any hope of certainty. There is always a joker in the pack to upset our carefully laid plans.

In ordinary awareness we use reason to interpret the information we absorb through the senses by a process of comparison and analysis. On occasions awareness sharpens and we can see not only the diversity of things but their unity as well. It is like seeing the jigsaw puzzle complete, with every piece in place, where before it was fragmented. This is not sub-rational, it is supra-rational. It is where opposites are reconciled, where black may well stand in opposition to white, but where the two are united as categories of colour.

With this tranquillity comes the tranquillity which eases pain.

We cannot give an amputee back his lost limb, we cannot

make black into white, any more than we can control which
cards we are dealt in a card game, but we can control the
way we react to these things. We can find peace in suffering
if we accept it, and with the knowledge that we have this
freedom it is then, in part, our own choice as to how much
we suffer. When pain is reduced from the global dimension
– why should this happen to me? Where will it end? How
much will I lose? – to the reality of each second's stab
of sensation, it is O.K. We can tolerate it.

When Bernadette first saw the vision of The Lady she
was afraid that she might be mad. Her mother told her
she was hallucinating and so, on her second visit, she
brought holy water and sprinkled it on the apparition. The
Lady smiled.

When we visited Lourdes we did not see The Lady. For
anyone to see such an apparition they must be possessed
of simplicity and directness almost impossible in this age
of sophistication. It is possible to be a visionary, to feel
the unity which transcends diversity, but to see a Person
standing and talking against the background of the "old
rock", the Massavieille, is way beyond most of us.

Bernadette saw The Lady and heard her speak. She
learned that her time on earth would be short and painful,
and she accepted all this. She was interrogated, not kindly,
by priests and police bcause the story of her vision was
attacting crowds to the town. Some of them touched and
drank the water from the spring she found, and were
healed.

When they saw there was money to be made, the police
and the clergy changed their tune. Wealth was invested
to re-direct the stream, to build baths, to build a beautiful
basilica so that, as now, thousands visit the grotto each day.
Thousands bathe in the water from the spring. Thousands
pray in consort, processing around the church.

We know nowadays that we cannot and shall not see The Lady – we would be locked up as mad people if we did – but we know and publicly profess our knowledge that there is more to life than the bare rocks, there is more than just the rational. We are not like Thomas, who had to put his hand in the wounds of Jesus before he could believe.

Lourdes is a demonstration of the third dimension, the dimension in which opposites are reconciled, where cripples can walk, where pain can be healed. It is a living demonstration of the wonder hidden beneath the prosaic stultification of life, the jewel in the lotus. On the way to Lourdes we sat in the airport for five hours, waiting for the plane. The *malades*, as the sick were called, were apprehensive. Some had obvious abnormalities, in others sickness was hard to recognize. One old man sat doubled-up in a wheelchair, he could hardly speak, he couldn't lift his head, he couldn't move his body. The men were the ones who looked after him – with such care and so gently. They held plastic cups to his lips, they spoke to him quietly, although he rarely responded. They never left him alone.

When at last we reached Lourdes the *malades* were taken straight to the hospital across the river. The Knights of Malta, whose pilgrimage it was, call them "Our Lords and Masters the sick, whom we are privileged to serve".

And it *was* a privilege. They trusted us, the helpers, with their lives, and all of us who worked with them felt this honour.

Twice during the week an international Mass was said in the Crypt, an enormous concrete building like an underground car park. Twenty-five thousand people attended, and the crypt was bursting with life and quiet movement. Helpers pull the sick in chariots called *voitures*. If the helpers are lucky two of them are assigned to each *voiture*, if not they heave and shove like pack horses.

Thousands of these carriages are parked in orderly rows in the crypt awaiting Mass. They have right of way in the town, even over cars, and in the crypt pedestrians move respectfully out of the way as the sick swing past.

My lady was a small, white-haired, lovely person called Lucy. She stared with large brown eyes out of a still, impassive face, like a small animal, until something touched her humour, when a wide, beaming smile irradiated her.

When we got to the crypt I was asked to look after two others as well, so I sat on the tow bar of the *voiture* ready for action if necessary. It proved not to be, but when I walked around the back of the carriages a hand reached up to me and one of them said, "You aren't leaving us, are you?" I realized then how alarming it must be and what courage it took to stay, unable to walk, surrounded by foreigners in a crowd of twenty-five thousand people, and underground.

The Mass was brilliantly choreographed, the altar lit by flickering candles, and a procession of 150 priests attending it. Monsieur Dechat conducted the singing with practised authority, and the whole enormous congregation obeyed him, singing in unison. When he wanted silence he made a sibilant, shushing noise into the microphone.

I saw behind me in the French contingent four people carrying a face like a dead flower. The body, what there was of it, was hidden beneath dark wrappings, and the white, beautifully structured, infinitely weary face, with its eyes closed – I never knew whether it was man or woman – was lifted gently into a chair where it rested, expressionless, until the priest came carrying the Eucharist. Then, wonderfully, for a second, the mouth opened and the eyes could see.

*

My second visit to Lourdes was with the Handicapped Children's Pilgrimage Trust, about which I knew nothing. I had met the secretary only once and it was his suggestion that I join the annual pilgrimage of two thousand five hundred children, of all ages and different religions.

We reached the airport at 7 a.m. in the cold of an English March morning, and were directed to the Administration Building. Coaches arrived and weary, excited bobble-hatted adults helped strangely abnormal children towards the loo after a night's drive from Leicester or Newcastle or anywhere in England, Wales, Scotland and Ireland. The bobble-hats and the accents indicated where they were from.

The strange thing was that the abnormalities were treated with such matter-of-factness that, after a while of sitting and watching, the abnormal became normal; the sight of a boy hobbling or a girl with little hands coming from out of her shoulders was not something to turn away from. This was the whole purpose of the pilgrimage.

We waited three hours for the plane. People were friendly but busy, they all had their jobs to do. One man sat by me and talked. He and his wife had brought their daughter first to the wrong building, then they weren't sure to which group they were assigned. I had seen the three walking up and down, the child was in a pushchair, about eight, with obvious brain damage. She could not move. Her face was impassive, her eyes, continually open, stared with no expression. She made no response to anything.

When I sat for half an hour on the coach taking us to the plane I found myself in the middle of a group of mixed children and helpers. One child, whom I couldn't see, was on her own, and was not assigned to anyone, so the group leader, John, sat next to her. He shared his attention between her and the other children of his group whom he was meeting for the first time, so I volunteered to sit next to the lonely child, who turned out to be the little girl in the wheelchair. She was propped in her seat, wrapped in a rug, staring forwards. There was no way of asking her, but I felt she must be very scared alone, surrounded by strangers, so I stroked her hand and talked, explaining every sound. I gave her orange juice to drink, frightened that I might be choking her but guided carefully by John, and moved the window curtain to protect her staring eyes from the warming sun. I was grieved to leave her when we reached the plane. Again I was reminded of the jewel in the lotus. We who are "normal" are clothed and covered by every sort of protective mechanism; we smile, we simper in shyness, we make jokes; we give instructions, we ask for names so that we can tabulate each other, we expect order in the proceedings around us. This child could neither see nor move. Although I talked to her continuously I did not know whether she heard. I held her hand, admiring the delicate, shell-like little nails. She was totally vulnerable. Her name was June, but to me she was a jewel without a name. Beneath the froth of our external presence we are all like this. While we hide behind our names we are separated from each other. We are "June", or Jane or Jack or Jim, with personality, with qualities to take pride in, with this or that or the other. This child was like you or me but stripped to the essence, glowing, because she had no option but to trust. She had no ego to defend. We are all like this when we die.

The next time I saw her was at the Blessing of the Sick which takes place every afternoon outside the Basilica. By this time I was with my own group, to whom I already felt a loyalty and great friendship. We were with our own children standing at the side, and I saw the little girl sitting in a wheelchair three rows from the front. I looked jealously at her assigned helper and was glad to see a kindly, smiling woman holding the chair.

Hundreds, thousands of people filled the square, prayers were recited in several languages, and after the verses a great rush of sound boomed around the church as they all sang.

Our group doctor stood behind me. I had never met him but I turned, grabbing his arm, and led him to a break in the crowd where he could see what I had seen. The little hands, drawn out from beneath the covers, beat feebly, gently, delicately in time with the music. When the sound stopped the hands lay still.

The doctor was excited too, and promised to talk to his colleague in June's group. Her parents probably knew already that she responded to music but maybe, just maybe, they didn't.

To me she had a name now. She responded. She was June.

The great thing about Lourdes – and this is why I want to work there, is that no one is tabulated out of existence. The sick are sick, but for the time they are there, they are released from their programming.

If you become sick you go to a doctor, and he tells you, "Yes, you have MS or cancer or arthritis or you are crippled and you will never walk again". He has to say this because we want to be able to foresee the future and we almost force him to predict it for us. Often he is unwilling to do so but we leave him with no option. He can only guess. He can use statistics, give the results of "controlled trials", but there is no objective truth either in statistics or research. We can only predict the "probable" result.

The prediction in itself becomes a form of conditioning. If we know the expected course of the disease, whatever it may be, we will tend to fulfil those expectations. If you expect to suffer great pain from a life-threatening disease you programme yourself to make that expectation a reality. I don't mean now that your pain is not "real", and I do not insult people by suggesting they are hypochondriacal, that their pains are imaginary. What I do say is that we add to our pain, we exacerbate it by our expectations and our fear.

One of the reasons why I stopped believing in Catholicism after my father's death was that I could no longer swallow such obviously unrational propositions as the virgin birth. I returned to Catholicism on the advice of a Buddhist when I realized that, if I wanted to understand Christianity, change and growth had to come from *me*, not from the religion.

One level on which the virgin birth can be understood and related to the way in which we lead our lives – otherwise what does it matter? – is that "virgin" means "without pre-conception". Every moment of time is like an incarnation, with limitless potential, when it is unclogged by prediction. When there is a pre-conception there can be no virginity. This is what real concentration is about: the mind moves through time, with time and in time. In that dimension there is no fear, there is no pre-conception. I dare to say it: there is no pain.

In Lourdes the Virgin, The Lady, is the important figure. St Bernadette was told, "I am the Immaculate Conception". On this second visit I began to see some reason why this is so important. I have never been very clear as to why the Immaculate Conception should matter so much to Catholics. I heard about it when I was a child, but being educated by nuns of that era I had no very clear idea of what a normal physical conception entailed, let alone an immaculate one.

Our concept of God seems beset by the Manichaean heresy. We say, "Thy Will be done", but when it is, we scream and shout in fear. We don't trust God. If we truly believed that He is good and omnipotent, as we pretend we do, we would see His will in everything. We would not be afraid. So often we see Him as a punishing God, almost a sadistic figure, waiting to strike us down the moment we transgress His unknowable Will. We know, or hope, that there must be a good side to Him, but He is like Janus, the God of two faces, sometimes kind, sometimes cruel.

The Lady is never held responsible for the sufferings of the world, but is always a figure of kindness, of compassion, intervening with her Son for us. She is one side of the coin only, the good, infinitely forgiving of the bad but not punitive.

We are wrong in thinking that God is a punishing God. That is a heresy, for God is good. It is we who punish ourselves and our children from one generation to the next. That is the greatest sadness of all: we blame God when we should be blaming ourselves.

Once in the pain relief unit I was asked to see a patient who had a terminal heart condition. Her only hope had been in having surgery, but this had not been successful. She had spent several hours in the theatre, and at one time had been declared clinically dead, but she recovered. When I saw her she was in great pain and knew that she must die very soon. She told me, and no one else, of the experience she had during her operation, though without making a big drama out of it.

She said that she knew she was dead and she met God. She said, "I call Him that because there is no other word to use, but I saw no person nor heard a real voice." This

God knew everything about her life and she said, "I knew what Julian of Norwich meant when she said, 'All shall be well, and all manner of things shall be well'. It was so peaceful. I asked, 'Why don't we know how simple it all is while we are alive?', but there was no answer."

She felt no pain until she knew she wanted to recover, because she wanted time to see that her children would be all right. Then she felt excruciating pain. She said she would never fear death again. She went home for the weekend, saw her children, sat alone by the fire waiting for the ambulance to bring her back, and died.

She was the lucky one. Most of us cannot reconcile the fact of suffering with the concept of a good God, but it is easier to do so with The Lady. She is not the Creator, so it isn't her fault that we suffer. Our trust in her is pure, and in her presence we don't try too hard to make sense of it all. We just rest in her compassion.

Then we are healed. We forget the doubts, the bartering with God – If I do this, will You do that? – we don't try to reduce God to a rational human level, we are encompassed by compassion. In that compassion everything is possible. Relief from suffering is possible. The strength to grasp the nettle of suffering, to face it and accept it is also within the bounds of possibility. That is why The Lady is the healing figure of Lourdes.

11

The Discipline of Adaptation

The human race has survived because not only do we have the power to adapt to the world around us but, through the development of technology, we have discovered ways of making the world adapt to us and to our wishes. When I was young if you felt cold you got chilblains. Now if you are cold you switch on the central heating. When I was young and wanted to go to Liverpool, the nearest big town, I had to travel across the Mersey. Literally – by boat, and it took a long time. Now I would drive through a tunnel under the river in twenty minutes.

Religious orders were founded in an attempt to restore the balance when the use of our powers to adapt the world to our convenience became distorted, when we began to get ideas above our station, when we became lazy. When novices asked to enter a religious order of any tradition, they knew that the rule of life in the monastery would not change to accommodate them. The routine of each day was planned, and very little allowance was made for the personal preference of individuals. Whether it was painful and unpleasant or not, the novices either learned to adapt and to change their emotional state, or they left.

It was a hard choice. In Christianity particularly the methodology of bringing about this change placed great emphasis on a militaristic type of discipline. The use of force in change, even *from* oneself *to* oneself, often changes only the outside activity – the deed. Christ demanded a change in the thought and the word as well. That is true adaptation, and the lack of it led to accusations of hypocrisy. It is comparatively easy to exhibit the outside signs of charity but sometimes they only mask a deep, hidden coldness or resentment.

The real methodology of how to change remains as it always has been, in the Christian tradition. It is there staring at us but we rarely see it. It is contained, as it is in every religious tradition, in the practice of the liturgy. In other traditions, particularly in the East, the methodology of change is usually more explicit. The techniques of Yoga and Zen lead students gradually towards an inner adaptation but, even so, some can study Yoga for years and learn only acrobatics.

Self-change is implicit in liturgical worship. Singing plain chant or reciting rhythmic mantras alters the rhythm of the breath and the rhythm of energy going to the brain. The long, controlled, gentle out-breath transforms angry, anxious hyper-activity into a state of receptive tranquillity. Gentle movements and periods of silence retrieve the mind from its constant preoccupation with the future, and with its futile attempts to control the exterior world by the force of the will.

One of the aims of communal chanting is to achieve synchronicity. Listening to the recital of the mantras or the daily office or the Islamic prayers makes it possible to assess whether the community is happy and in accord or not. You can tell by the degree of unison reached. There is no room for prima donnas, no place for the intrusive ego.

Sometimes the synchronicity is awe-inspiring. I discussed this with one of the Dominican sisters who said, "Oh yes. It is just like the 'bell tone' we looked for when I was rowing as a student at Oxford. When all the oars slip into the water together they make a special, distinctive sound – a bell tone. It is the same when we reach unison in reciting the office." Another told me that the irritations and upsets which occur in any close community tended to be ironed out and forgotten after joining together to recite the liturgy. It is another means of reaching the emotional control discussed in chapter 3.

We may read holy books admonishing us to surrender to the will of God; to realize that we are all equally children of God; that our ambition, greed for self-aggrandisement, and fear of losing individual power is at the heart of all our suffering. We can take this on board intellectually, and the knowledge rests easily in one of the layers of the brain, but when called on to sing the office or chant a mantra or recite communal prayers we cannot rest unchanged. We cannot remain a self-idolizing, spoiled child. We have to become one of the many children of God, adapting thinking, speaking and doing in order to synchronize with each other and to find tranquillity and harmony in so doing.

Some religious understand all this. I have talked to eminent leaders from various traditions and they do not differ. If a religious, from whatever part of the world, is happy, he has learned to adapt. If he is unhappy, he has not.

Behavioural psychologists try to teach methods of adaptation by using mechanistic methods of conditioning. At one time in America they even experimented by inserting electrodes into the brains of prisoners to change their response, so that, even in intolerable circumstances, they felt happy. The end does not justify the means. When I once thought of doing a degree in psychology the humanistic psychologists warned me to keep away from the experimental psychologists and their works, telling me that even *they* disapproved of what went on under the banner of experimental science.

The mechanism of the totality of the human person is

too complex, too subtle to benefit by forced, invasive alteration. Change brought about voluntarily by oneself is a gradual transformation, incorporating body, mind and spirit. Change brought about by an invasive violation cannot be of benefit.

The major disciplines for such a gradual, conscious, self-adaptation are to be found in the set of formularies contained within the public worship of each of the great traditions.

Because I was "a cradle Catholic" my most direct experience came from going to the Mass. When I had left Catholicism, one of the reasons why Marco Pallis, a Buddhist, advised me to return to it, was because, he said, my roots were implanted in the religion of my birth: the deep, subconscious psychic awareness of the sacramental life was already a part of me. It made sense and saved time to take advantage of this, while at the same time learning from him about the universality of all the traditions. He called me a Buddhist-flavoured Catholic, and at his death the Tibetan ceremonies were another aspect of the requiem I already knew.

I started going to Mass at an early age, and from the beginning, it was an unwelcome chore. I rarely admitted to this because we were supposed to be filled with holy thoughts and unctions. I was not, I was bored out of my mind. I counted every candle sloping up one side of the altar and then every candle sloping down the other. I added them up, subtracted them, multiplied the result. I dropped the tin box containing my rosary beads in the middle of a young priest's sermon, upsetting his train of thought to such an extent that he had to stop. I was renowned, as a child too young to be punished, for having said loudly during a preacher's dramatic pause, "What is that man talking about?" Escaping afterwards from the dark church into freedom and the light of day was the best thing about it.

At boarding school we seemed to spend most of our waking life in the chapel, but in contrast to the austerity of our living conditions, I recognized something of the beauty of the Mass – the music; the candles flaring, outlined in the darkness; the rhythm of the Latin responses; it was the only place where I was allowed to be alone inside myself, unobserved, unquestioned, anonymous.

When my father died I was fifteen and wanted to find reasons for everything, including death. There seemed no rationality in either the Mass or Catholicism, so I left both. Watching the people in church bobbing up and down as they genuflected, shuffling up to the altar for Communion, yawning visibly during the sermon, fumbling for money for the collection, knowing that at least some of them were as bored as I was, made the whole process seem like a ludicrous waste of time.

After wandering in the wilderness for some time I met Marco, who told me to attend the sacraments because that was the most important aspect of Catholicism, and to read Meister Eckhart. I have already written about this in the introduction to my book *Meister Eckhart: The Man from whom God hid Nothing*.

When I told Marco that I actively disliked going to Mass, he said, ''Your emotions are irrelevant. Keep on going to the Eucharist and, eventually, you may be privileged to learn what it is about.'' So I did.

I had no idea of how helpful it would become. Now I go to Mass every day not from piety or duty but because I *need* this discipline. But it was only when I applied what I had learned in relaxation, learning to live *with* my body instead of just *inside* it, that I began to get an inkling of what could really become available to me.

I began to wonder why, during Mass, my body was guided very specifically and carefully through a series of movements. There was nothing haphazard about it: these movements were choreographed. I became aware of the sloppy way in which I responded: the clumsy, mechanistic way I knelt and genuflected, then stood or sat; the self-conscious way I walked towards the altar with all the others, unco-ordinated, staring around, shuffling robots more than human animals. My relaxation teacher had been a dancer, and I had learned from her how, in movement, the mind learns from the body, and how controlled spontaneity is the essence of artistic creation.

The purpose of all religious traditions is to learn to adapt, to harmonize with the world around us, to learn to understand, to accept and to overcome the pain of living.

I went to Mass knowing that it would not be entertaining – I had heard it all many times before – yet unaware of what other purpose there might be. I even flirted with the idea that God might be pleased at my attendance and so make life a little easier for me – make the sun shine for sports day, or make my school teachers tolerant of my faults. But I found out that this was a little too naive – and it didn't work, anyway.

Eventually I found that participating in the Mass is a healing, transforming, very practical process. The whole form and the structure move towards that end. Attending Mass as a watcher, observing and listening to the priest, expecting to be entertained, is not enough. Participation is of the essence, but, as in medicine, the healing of the Mass is holistic: it engages the body – in stillness and in movement – the mind, and the spirit.

This participation should not, however, be confused with the hyperactivity which sometimes takes place in a family or children's Mass – constant noisy singing, indiscriminate use of musical instruments; everyone leaping around praising the Lord.

Healing is a part of learning, and in order to learn we must first listen. Where there is constant activity and no silence there can be no learning. There is a place for the overflow of enthusiasm, for the Mass as entertainment, but I suspect that it appeals more to confused adults than to children. Children have endless opportunities to express exuberance, and don't need to do so in church.

When I returned to the Mass after some years of absence I looked on it with new eyes. At one stage the priest says, "Relieve us from all anxiety." He doesn't say, "Take away all the causes of anxiety", but he says, "Take away the anxiety itself". All that I have learned about pain control is working towards just this – reconciliation of opposites, tranquillity, finding peace even in pain. It centres round the Christ who walked forward to face a horrible death when He could easily have escaped it by running away.

I looked to find out what the movements of the Mass did to change *me* rather than how I performed *them* and what they looked like from the outside. If unclenching my hands changed my state of mind from anger to comparative peace, what did the movements of the Mass do?

I found that sitting upright on the benches ideally suited for this posture made active concentration more possible. When I slumped, my mind started to wander and to daydream. There is no picture of the Buddha sitting in a lax position, always his back is upright. When I joined a group for Tibetan meditation we sat cross-legged on the floor for an hour in complete stillness. If our backs had been crooked and the weight unevenly distributed we would have had cramps and spasms of all sorts, or we would have fallen asleep.

The Christian tradition fell into heresy when it saw the body as an evil. It sometimes falls into heresy now when it sees the body as something to be indulged, where the positive value of pain is disregarded and we are told we have the right to live pain-free.

Attending Mass is the way I achieve a daily baseline of tranquillity, without which I would be lost. There is nothing sentimental about it: I go to Mass because I know that, if I work at it in the right way, when I come out I will be relieved of all anxiety. I will be happy.

Professional religious in the Christian tradition return to the church maybe four or five times in the day for the daily office – lauds, terce, sext, none, vespers and compline – so that they may come back to this baseline of tranquillity if they have strayed away from it.

In the tradition of Islam the same discipline is required of all worshippers, not only of the professed contemplatives. They pray at first light, at sunrise, again at midday when the sun is at its zenith and casts no shadow, and again at sunset.

They stand with shoulders touching to form a solid line while the Koran is recited. They bow down from the waist so that the back of the head and the waist are parallel to the ground, praying for all animal creation. Then, after coming back to the vertical, they prostrate saying, "Glory to God the most high". They crouch in the foetal position, physically reduced in size to a nothing under the ray of transcendence. They raise their hands, palms upwards, making themselves both vulnerable and accepting. Whatever the work they may be doing, it is stopped at these times for the prayer which is a renewal of the harmony and the unity of mind, body and spirit.

I found that people in the Orthodox Church prostrate in the same way, and so do the Tibetan Buddhists. In every tradition there seems to be some form of prostration. In the Dominican order the friars used to prostrate whenever they had given offence, but theirs was a full prostration where they stretched out flat on the floor. It has more effect than a spoken apology. They prostrated, too, when they were ordained and became "dead to the world". Tibetan pilgrims sometimes prostrate continuously, measuring their length on the ground and then standing, as a means of moving towards their goal. The words of self-abasement are not enough – the veneration of God has to be expressed in actions too.

In the Catholic Church it is customary to genuflect, to go down on one knee and then to stand again, a sort of mini prostration. It is the beginning. Before the words begin we go back into a deeper stage and talk with our bodies, kneeling is a recognition, an affirmation, of our need to learn. Soon after the innovations of Vatican II, when the practices of Catholicism were modernized, a young novice said to me, "I could never genuflect or kneel in prayer. I would feel like Uriah Heep, as though I was crawling to God instead of seeing Christ as my brother." No matter what our modern educationalists may say, no one can learn if they don't first accept the superior knowledge of their teacher. The traditional respect paid to a teacher is because he knows more than his pupil. In this context talking is not enough: we have to kneel before the immensity of creation, admitting that we don't understand it and that we need to learn.

In kneeling, as in prostration, we begin to separate out from each other; we begin to face our own aloneness, our own problems, our own pain, our own God. In sitting we are mobile, the head can turn, the hands can move, but the balance of the kneeling body brings it to stillness and to a positive sense of isolation.

This first part of the Mass helps in the transition from the outer, where all the world's a stage and we are only actors, to the inner self, wherein we are alone and with no audience. The church is an oasis in the desert of our daily life, the demands of which are left outside the door. The Muslims leave their shoes but we Christians have no symbol for this. Inside the church there are no demands, and we are free to change direction from the pre-occupation with day-to-day affairs to awareness of the tranquillity and harmony within ourselves.

The form of the Mass, the quiet gestures of the priest and the response of the people, all lead away from mechanical living to the world of art where God communicates Himself. The sign of the Cross, where the right hand touches the head or the mind in the name of the Father; the heart, the body, in the name of the Son; then the shoulders in the name of the Spirit, brings the truth of the Trinity into live reach of the body – the head and the heart and the Spirit which energizes them.

The Confiteor, where we confess our sins, has something in common with the act of leaving the shoes outside. We confess our corporate sins because they are a nuisance, a stupidity, a hindrance in the search for peace. We put them away right at the beginning and we can then forget them.

It is significant that we do not make any individual confession. There is no call for great heart-searching, which may bring with it the danger of measuring ourselves against perfection and let in the real threat to tranquillity, the real source of pain, the ego. Sins can become a source of pride: "I really am so perfect but just look at what I have done." We all sin. Every priest must know how boringly similar our plight is, from his experiences in the confessional. It is best to say, "OK, we have all sinned. Let us accept that we all need help and get on with it."

The sins, like the shoes, are left outside the door.

When the priest reads the gospel we stand. Moving from sitting to standing without losing concentration, without shuffling and fidgeting, happens easily when breathing-in is extended and lifts the body up. The movement becomes, in the words of Nicholas of Cusa, "Stillness drawn out in an orderly series".

Standing still to listen with the head erect, as it is meant to be, and the arms hanging loosely by the sides, is a vulnerable postion to adopt. Our primitive ancestors knew better than to leave the back unprotected, and the same sense of unease is instinctive in us. But we *need* to make ourselves vulnerable if we are to stir from the torpor of our normal life and alter our state of consciousness. We don't have to be scholars to understand what Christ was saying, but we do have to make the connections which relate his words to the way in which we conduct our lives. We do need to concentrate, to hear the familiar words as if they were always new, in the hope that sometime they may permeate through all the dross clogging up our minds and make us change, giving us peace, transforming our pain.

That is the blessing used continually during the Mass: "The peace of the Lord be always with you." And the answer: "And also with you." We ask for it all the time but the saying of the words can become so mechanical that we don't even hear what we want for ourselves. When we are at peace we are free from pain.

Making the body vulnerable, unsafe yet standing erect and deliberately relaxed and unafraid, makes us vulnerable, too, to the words of the Gospel. We are more likely then to work at increasing our understanding. We are not talking here about specific Roman Catholic doctrine, we are talking about wholeness, about the three-in-one which unifies us. And talking itself is not enough.

We are talking about listening, and if the body is concentrated, relaxed and still, so is the mind and so is the spirit. When the priest delivers the sermon he talks, giving his own opinions, as a man. He chooses his own words, links his own thoughts, faces us as one of uṣ – and we judge him accordingly.

The kindness and the courtesy extended by the people to the priest is limitless, and is one of the recurring miracles. He may stutter or stumble; on many occasions the thoughts he expresses are stereotyped, and with neither profundity nor interest. At times the people gently go to sleep, Mothers chide their children into quiescence; eyes wander round the church, noting a neighbour's new hat, looking for solace in the stained glass in the windows, wondering how long it will be before the pub will open or the roast be baked.

People are not stupid. Whether we have been educated or not has nothing to do with our capacity to understand our misery. Intelligent people are no nearer the answer to pain than anyone else.

The difference is shown in the choice of words. Educated people express themselves more subtly because they have more words available in their armoury. If the priest, instead of dredging up platitudes each week which he may think suitable for an unsophisticated parish audience, tried to translate for them current theological thinking, the result might be surprising.

A nineteen-year-old tyre fitter was detailed by his devout mother to attend a lecture given by an eminent theologian on the *via negativa*. The lecture was good. Afterwards the boy said, ''I wish my brother had been here to hear this. He wouldn't spend his time during Mass playing noughts and crosses at the back of the church if we got stuff like this.'' The brother was sixteen.

After the gospel we stand to affirm our belief. It doesn't

matter too much if that belief is shaky – there is not one of us who has not at some stage said, "Is there really a God or am I conning myself?" There would be something strange about a belief which knew nothing of disbelief. It would be like a world without pain. It is through pain that we learn about peace. It is often through facing disbelief that we learn about belief. Accept disbelief and let it go, until you relax and become receptive to belief.

The next stage of the Mass is about the Eucharist. By this time, having left the cares of the world, having acknowledged and put aside our sins and our stupidities, having heard the priest speak to us, and having affirmed our belief, however shaky, we should be, we try to be, ready to move from pre-occupation with the body and the mind to recognition of the spirit.

By this time the body should be relaxed and still, the mind should be concentrated, aware of each moment of time touching like a drop of rain or a beam of light. If this is not so, if we are still fragmented and in pain, then we have not worked hard enough at the changing process, at the preliminary preparation; we have not used the disciplines made available to us.

At the heart of our being and deeply, in every thing we do, is the element of mystery. When we are awake, and remember that for a third of our life we are *not* awake, we are in a state of conscious awareness of ourselves and of the world around. We are aware but we don't understand. We cannot. All the questions – Why am I alive? – Why am I in pain? – Why am I unhappy? – Why am I happy? – are all unanswered. We don't know where we are going or where we come from, our rational understanding is severely limited.

At the Offertory of the Mass, bread and wine are brought to the altar by the people, to be consecrated and offered up to God. In rational terms this is quite crazy: there is no God whom we can see or touch; the altar is just a table; the priest is an ordinary man dressed up in grand clothes; the bread and wine is just bread and wine.

But if we are to make sense of the Mass, just as in making sense of pain, we must let go of thought, forget the whys and wherefores, and focus on what IS. When you let go of the protection of thought a small, little gap appears in the layers of confusion, and the possibility breaks through it like the gold of sunlight, that harmony within oneself and with the world around and the people in it does exist; that the pain of living, be it physical or mental, is a paradox. Physical pain is inflicted upon us, but still we have the choice either to collude with this infliction or not.

It is not for me to write about the theology of the Eucharist. All I can say is that at one time I thought it was a crazy game where the priests conned the people and they willingly colluded. It was the opium of the people and the bread and butter of the priests. But Marco, the Buddhist, was right. After working and working at it I know that it is not a con. Every time I go to Mass I learn more – not about how to be ''holy'' or how to deceive myself into thinking that everything is sweetness and light and that pain does not exist. I learn how to transform pain. There was a time when I could hardly walk and had great pain in my leg. Going down the hill to Mass was killing, but walking up it afterwards was no problem.

Many years ago I read a translation of Lao Tse in which he said, ''Every stick has two ends''. One end of the stick could be called ''pleasure'', one end could be ''pain''. But as well as the two ends, there is the wholeness of the stick encompassing both.

Although the discipline of adaptation is there for the taking in the Christian liturgy, it is used with much more

169

respect and conscious awareness in other traditions. Muslims pray with their whole being, body, mind and spirit, and the results show. At the London Mosque I was asked whether I was a visitor, and I was welcomed, instructed, even fed, with a warmth I have never seen in a Christian church, be it Catholic, Anglican or Orthodox. Muslims move, in prayer, with a grace which demonstrates the respect they have for their own bodies.

We have to take what help we can, where and when we can get it. Above all we need to learn. Forget all about hierarchies or about competition. Forget all about comparing yourself with other people, what they have done or what they might think of you. Only you can solve the problem of your pain. Only you can teach yourself to face the world without fear. In deep tranquillity.

TAPES

Details of the following tapes are available from:
Ursula Fleming Tapes,
P.O. Box No. 1902,
London NW3 2UF

Relax to Ease Pain
Relax to Concentrate
Relax to Ease Stress
Relax to Pray

Half Way
Jim Thompson

We all have to face the changes that middle age brings. Jim Thompson shows how this can be a time of growth, development and change for the better in all areas of our life.

"... a warm, stimulating book ..."
John King, Church of England Newspaper

Now and For Ever
Anne Townsend

"A well-researched, highly relevant book on all aspects of marriage today ... Amidst the current spate of books on marriage, this one stands apart, deserving a place on the best sellers list."
Susan Rimmer, Church of England Newspaper

Mother Teresa: Contemplative in the Heart of the World
Angelo Devananda

This book focuses upon the spirituality which has inspired the wonderful work of Mother Teresa among the poor and dying, consisting mainly of long passages of her own words.

Also available in Fount Paperbacks

BOOKS BY C. S. LEWIS

Reflections on the Psalms

'Absolutely packed with wisdom. It is clearly the fruit of very much reflection . . . upon one's own darkness of spirit, one's own fumbling and grasping in the shadows of prayer or of penitence.'

Trevor Huddleston

Miracles

'This is a brilliant book, abounding in lucid exposition and illuminating metaphor.'

Charles Davey, The Observer

The Problem of Pain

'Written with clarity and force, and out of much knowledge and experience.'

Times Literary Supplement

Surprised by Joy

'His outstanding gift is clarity. You can take it at two levels, as straight autobiography, or as a kind of spiritual thriller, a detective's probing of clue and motive . . .'

Isabel Quigley, Sunday Times

Fount Paperbacks

Fount is one of the leading paperback publishers of religious books and below are some of its recent titles.

- [ ] FRIENDSHIP WITH GOD David Hope £2.95
- [ ] THE DARK FACE OF REALITY Martin Israel £2.95
- [ ] LIVING WITH CONTRADICTION Esther de Waal £2.95
- [ ] FROM EAST TO WEST Brigid Marlin £3.95
- [ ] GUIDE TO THE HERE AND HEREAFTER
        Lionel Blue/Jonathan Magonet £4.50
- [ ] CHRISTIAN ENGLAND (1 Vol) David Edwards £10.95
- [ ] MASTERING SADHANA Carlos Valles £3.95
- [ ] THE GREAT GOD ROBBERY George Carey £2.95
- [ ] CALLED TO ACTION Fran Beckett £2.95
- [ ] TENSIONS Harry Williams £2.50
- [ ] CONVERSION Malcolm Muggeridge £2.95
- [ ] INVISIBLE NETWORK Frank Wright £2.95
- [ ] THE DANCE OF LOVE Stephen Verney £3.95
- [ ] THANK YOU, PADRE Joan Clifford £2.50
- [ ] LIGHT AND LIFE Grazyna Sikorska £2.95
- [ ] CELEBRATION Margaret Spufford £2.95
- [ ] GOODNIGHT LORD Georgette Butcher £2.95
- [ ] GROWING OLDER Una Kroll £2.95

All Fount Paperbacks are available at your bookshop or newsagent, or they can be ordered by post from Fount Paperbacks, Cash Sales Department, G.P.O. Box 29, Douglas, Isle of Man. Please send purchase price plus 22p per book, maximum postage £3. Customers outside the UK send purchase price, plus 22p per book. Cheque, postal order or money order. No currency.

NAME (Block letters) _____

ADDRESS_____

_____

_____